VEGAN SLOW COOKER COOKBOOK

Easy and Healthy Meals for Busy People

(Amazing, Healthy, and Easy Vegan Slow Cooker Recipes for Everyone)

Stephanie Nowak

Published by Sharon Lohan

© **Stephanie Nowak**

All Rights Reserved

Vegan Slow Cooker Cookbook: Easy and Healthy Meals for Busy People (Amazing, Healthy, and Easy Vegan Slow Cooker Recipes for Everyone)

ISBN 978-1-990334-34-4

All rights reserved. No part of this guide may be reproduced in any form without permission in writing from the publisher except in the case of brief quotations embodied in critical articles or reviews.

Legal & Disclaimer

The information contained in this book is not designed to replace or take the place of any form of medicine or professional medical advice. The information in this book has been provided for educational and entertainment purposes only.

The information contained in this book has been compiled from sources deemed reliable, and it is accurate to the best of the Author's knowledge; however, the Author cannot guarantee its accuracy and validity and cannot be held liable for any errors or omissions. Changes are periodically made to this book. You must consult your doctor or get professional medical advice before using any of the suggested remedies, techniques, or information in this book.

Table of contents

Part 1 1
Introduction 2
Vegan Guidelines 3
Benefits of Slow Cookers 5
Slow Cookers 101 7
Soups 10
Corn Chowder 10
Cannellini Bean And Kale Soup 12
Potato And Leek Soup 13
Minestrone Soup 14
Pasta And Grains 16
Mac And "Cheese" With A Twist 16
Sweet Potato And Spinach Cannelloni 18
Quinoa Pilaf 20
Pearl Barley With Broccoli And Spinach 21
Mushroom And Pea Risotto 22
Stuff It! 23
Stuffed Tomatoes 23
Stuffed Bell Peppers 24
Stuffed Zucchini Boats 25
Cabbage Rolls 26
Stews And Chili 28
Chinese Hot Pot 28
Butternut Squash And Coconut Chili 29
Super Easy Black Beans 31

Portuguese Fava Beans 32

Easy Italian Lentils 33

Creamy Sweet Potato Stew 34

Classic Veggie Chili 35

Curries 36

Indian-Inspired Cauliflower And Garbanzo Bean Curry 36

Cashew Cream Veggie Korma 38

Malaysian Laksa 40

Breads 42

Vegan Egg Replacer 42

Healthy Banana And Walnut Loaf 42

Corn Bread 44

Rosemary Bread 46

Desserts 48

Rice Pudding 48

Cranberry And Peach Crumble 49

Pumpkin Pudding 50

Stewed Rhubarb And Strawberry Sauce 51

Chocolate Peanut Butter Cake 52

Soups & Stews 54

Curried Vegetables And Chickpea Stew 54

Indian Spiced Lentils 57

'Cream' Of Mushroom Soup 59

White Bean Soup 61

Chickpea, Butternut Squash And Red Lentil Stew 63

Crockpot Thai Coconut Soup 65

Potato Zucchini Soup 67

Butternut Squash And Parsnip Soup 69
African Peanut Stew 70
Hearty Vegetable And Bean Soup 72
Main Courses 73
Quinoa Jambalaya With Tempeh 75
Slow Cooker Chili 76
Root Veggie Barley Risotto 77
Crock Pot Bbq 'Beef' 79
Homemade Bbq Sauce 80
Crock Pot Quinoa With Vegetables 81
Vegan Crock Pot Tacos 82
Vegan Brown Rice Mexican Bowl 83
Vegan Crock Pot Polenta Lasagna 86
'Cheese' Sauce 87
Slow Cooker Spaghetti 88
Side Dishes 91
Slow Cooker Potatoes With Garlic And Rosemary 91
Slow Cooked Apples and Butternut Squash 92
Slow Cooked Collard Greens 93
Slow-Cooked Baked Beans 95
Broccoli Toasted With Garlic And Hazelnuts 96
Part 2 98
1. Chili 99
2. Black Bean And Quinoa Soup 101
3. Leek And Potato Soup 103
4. Minestrone Soup 104
5. Lentil And Barley Soup 106

6. Split Pea Soup 109
7. Black Bean Soup 111
8. Vegan Ratatouille 113
9. Sweet And Spicy Curry 115
10. Bean And Spinach Enchiladas 117
11. Mushroom Stroganoff 119
12. Lentil Taco Filling 121
13. Fajitas Filling 123
14. Non-Fried Refried Beans 124
15. Slow Cooker Spicy Chickpeas 126
16. Mediterranean Vegetables With Beans 128
17. Sweet Potato Risotto 130
18. Red Beans And Barley 132
19. Slow Cooker Greens 134
20. Winter Stew 136
21. Stuffed Zucchini 138
22. Almond Barley Casserole 140
23. Pineapple Barbecue Tofu 142
24. Wild Rice 144
25. Chai Pear Applesauce 145
26. Maple Brown Sugar Oatmeal 147
27. Lemon Blueberry Cake 149
28. Coconut Rice Pudding 151
29. Scalloped Peaches 153
30. Cinnamon Applesauce 154
Southern Style Beets 157
Summer Zucchini 157

Greek Style Eggplant	157
Dinner Vegetable Medley	158
Italian Stewed Tomatoes	159
Slow Cooked Artichokes	159
Stuffed Peppers	160
Barbecue Tofu	161
Teriyaki Tofu	161
White Beans and Sun Dried Tomatoes	162
Slow Cooker Ravioli	163
Three Bean Italian Cassoulet	163
Barley Casserole	164
Meatless Sloppy Joes	165
Southern Chickpeas and Grits	166
Lemon Pepper Tofu	166
No Beans Refried Beans	167
Carrot Pudding	168
Orange Pecan Carrots	168
German Cole Slaw	169
Cauliflower Mash	169
Brocolli with Toasted Hazelnuts	170
Teriyaki Broccoli and Mushrooms	170
Honey Dijon Brussels Sprouts	171
Lemon Pepper Brussels Sprouts	171
Garlic Lemon Asparagus	172
Winter Root Vegetable Medley	172
Smashed Turnips	173
Baked Sweet Potatoes	174

Caramel Glazed Sweet Potatoes ... 174
Slow Cooker Corn on the Cob ... 175
Summer Garlic Green Beans ... 175
Fast and Easy Slow Cooker Rice ... 176
Cajun Beans and Rice ... 176
Sweet Pineapple Baked Beans ... 177
Scalloped Potatoes ... 177
Vegan Slow Cooker Fudge ... 178
Bananas Foster ... 179
Honey Glazed Pears ... 180
Southern Cherry Jubilee ... 180
Walnut Strawberry Surprise ... 181
Hawaiian Tapioca Pudding ... 181
Berry Mint Medley ... 182
Chocolate Peanut Butter Cake ... 182
Simple Rice Pudding ... 183
Slow Cooker Apple Cobbler ... 184
Georgia Peach Cobbler ... 185
Crustless Pumpkin Pie ... 186
Apple Pudding Can Cake ... 186
Cherry Cobbler ... 187
Simple Marinara Sauce ... 187

Part 1

Introduction

Whether you're new to vegan eating, have been vegan for years, or are even just looking to eat more veggies, you're going to love the recipes in this book. No matter what diet you follow, everyone agrees that it's essential to eat more plant-based foods.

However, let's face it: sometimes vegan recipes can be a pain and involve heaps of prep. Well, not these recipes! By using your slow cooker, you'll be able to get maximum taste out of simple ingredients and – better yet – you'll be amazed just how easy it can be.

I'm sure you're going to love all of the delicious meals in this book, including soups, stews, chili, curries, breads, risotto, pasta, desserts and much more! Not only that, your friends and family are sure to love the dishes as well. Ready to get started?

Vegan Guidelines

The vegan diet excludes all animal products. Unlike vegetarians, vegans do not eat eggs, dairy products, or other ingredients derived from animals. Contrary to popular belief, a vegan diet isn't at all restrictive or limited. In fact, it offers you the scope to include a wide range of healthy plant-based foods that provide all the essential nutrients you need. Check out some of the allowed foods:

1. Vegetables
2. Fruits
3. Seeds and nuts
4. Vegan breads and pastas
5. Grains
6. Vegetable oils
7. Legumes and beans
8. Soy and nut milks
9. Soy products like tofu and tempeh
10. Maple syrup and other plant-based syrups

Some Cautions
While everyone needs to make their own dietary choices, there are a few foods to watch out for if you want to follow a strict vegan diet. These include:

1. **Breads and pastas**. These need to be checked carefully to make sure they're free from eggs, whey and other milk products.

2. **Dressings and sauces**. Check the ingredients carefully to make sure they don't include dairy products or eggs.

3. **Honey**. This obviously comes from bees, and so is not consumed by strict vegans.

4. **Gelatin**. While we all know Jell-O has gelatin, which is an animal product, don't forget that marshmallows and other sweets also often contain it.

5. **Sugar**. It's important to be aware that the sugar refining process often uses bone char! It is possible to buy vegan-safe sugar in some stores, otherwise alternatives include palm sugar, maple syrup and other plant-derived syrups, such as rice syrup, and sweeteners such as stevia.

6. **Beer**. This can also be processed using animal products.

Benefits of Slow Cookers

Vegan slow cooker recipes have heaps of benefits. Some of the reasons they're great include that vegan slow cooker meals are:

1. **Stress-free**. Slow cookers are convenient and make life easy. You don't need to slave away over a hot stove for hours on end. Instead, you can put your meal on before you go to work and by the time you come home, your dinner's ready.

2. **Safe**. You can leave your slow cooker unattended for hours without any risk of burning your meal, or your home!

3. **Healthy**. When you see just how easy it is to prepare healthy slow cooker meals, you won't be tempted to pick up fast food or heat up a TV dinner.

4. **Cheap**. By not getting take-out or buying prepared meals, you'll save some serious cash.

5. **Cheap!** Because slow cookers use long cooking times, you can easily make use of cheap ingredients like carrots and potatoes to prepare mouthwatering dishes.

6. **Bulk**. You can cook extra and keep the leftovers for lunch or freeze them for another day.

7. **Easy entertaining**. Slow-cooked dishes are simply wonderful when you're cooking for large groups of people or preparing holiday meals. Not only do they take the stress out of preparing for holidays like Christmas, but slow cookers also free up your oven and stove.

Slow Cookers 101

If you're new to slow cooking, here are some essential guidelines to help you get started straight away.

Size Matters
Slow cookers come in different sizes, so you'll need to think about what'll best suit you. If you have 3 to 4 people in your home, then a 4-quart slow cooker will meet your needs. On the other hand, if you have a larger family, a 6-quart model is ideal. Of course, if you like to cook in bulk to have extra on hand for lunches or to freeze, take this into consideration and up the size.

Shape
While slow cookers come in round, oval and rectangular shapes, I personally think the round ones are easier to clean and are better for making cakes and bread. Of course, this is up to you.

Placement
Although the basic idea behind slow cooking is to leave the cooker unattended for long periods of times, you should still ensure it's located several inches away from the wall or any other electrical appliances. After all, they do still generate a bit of heat during the cooking process.

Don't Fill it Up!

Try not to get too excited and fill your slow cooker all the way up to the rim. Instead, your cooker should be only half to three-quarters full so that the ingredients get enough space to cook well and release their flavors. Each slow cooker is different, so make sure you check the manufacturer's guidelines.

Keep that Lid On
Slow cookers work by building the temperature up and then continuing the cooking at this stable temperature. For this reason, most recipes require you to snugly fit the slow cooker lid and leave it on. Don't be tempted to keep taking the lid off! You should only open the lid if the recipe requires adding more ingredients after a particular cooking time.

Safely Cooking Beans
Some beans, including kidney beans, contain a toxin called phytohaemagglutinin. Normally this toxin is killed at high temperatures but some special precautions need to be taken when cooking dried beans in your slow cooker. Follow these safety steps:

1. Soak the beans in water overnight
2. Discard the soaking water and rinse the beans
3. Place the beans in a pan, cover with water and boil on the stove for 10 minutes
4. You can then safely proceed with the recipe in your slow cooker

A quicker and simpler option is to use canned beans, which don't require any of the above steps. The recipes in this book call for canned beans, but you can substitute dry beans, providing you follow the safety instructions given above.

Use Your Timer
Most modern slow cookers have a timer, so take advantage of it.

Instructions
Don't forget to read your slow cooker manual and follow the manufacturer's instructions.

Happy slow cooking!

Soups

Corn Chowder

Serves 6 to 8

Ingredients

3 large potatoes, diced
20 oz. frozen sweet corn (2 packets)
5 cups vegetable stock
1 tablespoon olive oil
1 yellow onion, diced
2 cloves garlic, minced
1 teaspoon paprika
1 teaspoon dried oregano
1 bay leaf
Salt and pepper to taste

Method

1. Heat the oil in a skillet and sauté the onion until soft and translucent.
2. Add the garlic and paprika and sauté for a further 30 seconds.
3. Put the sautéed onion, garlic and paprika into your slow cooker along with all the other ingredients. Mix well. Cook on low for 6-8 hours.
4. Before serving, remove the bay leaf, and mash with a potato masher or blend with a stick blender. Or

leave as is and enjoy it chunky! Season to taste with salt and pepper.

Cannellini Bean And Kale Soup

Serves 6 to 8

Ingredients

2 (15 oz. each) cans cannellini beans with juice
1 (14.5 oz.) can tomatoes, diced with juice
2 cups kale, washed and finely chopped
6 cups vegetable stock
2 tablespoons olive oil
2 medium onions, finely chopped
2 teaspoons garlic, minced
2 teaspoons dried basil
2 teaspoons dried marjoram
2 teaspoons dried thyme

Method

1. Heat the olive oil in a skillet and sauté the onions until translucent.
2. Add the garlic and sauté for another minute. Turn off the heat.
3. Puree the cannellini beans and juice in your food processor.
4. Put the garlic and onions into the slow cooker, along with the pureed cannellini beans and all the other ingredients.
5. Cook for 4 hours on high heat or for 6 to 8 hours on low heat.

Potato And Leek Soup

Serves 4

Ingredients

2 leeks, roughly chopped (make sure you wash them well!)
3 medium potatoes, diced
3 cups vegetable stock
1 cup pure unsweetened almond milk (or soy milk)
1 yellow onion, diced
2 cloves garlic, minced
1 bay leaf
Salt and pepper to taste

Method

1. Put all the ingredients into your slow cooker and stir to combine.
2. Cook on low for 6 hours or high for 4 hours.
3. Before serving, remove the bay leaf, blend with a stick blender and season to taste with salt and pepper.

Minestrone Soup

Serves 6

Ingredients

2 carrots, chopped
2 celery stalks, chopped
2 zucchinis, chopped
1 large onion, chopped
3 cups vegetable broth
1 (28 ounce) can crushed tomatoes
1 (15 ounce) can cranberry beans, drained and rinsed
3 garlic cloves, minced
1 tablespoon dried parsley
1 1/2 teaspoons dried oregano
1 teaspoon dried basil
1/2 teaspoon freshly ground black pepper

To serve
1 cup elbow macaroni
1/2 cup grated vegan parmesan
Fresh sweet basil leaves

Method

1. Place all the ingredients into the slow cooker.
2. Cook on low heat for 6 to 8 hours.
3. Before serving, cook the elbow macaroni on the stove top in salted water for around 8-10 minutes, or until al dente.

4. Stir the macaroni through the minestrone and garnish with vegan parmesan and fresh basil leaves.

Pasta And Grains

Mac And "Cheese" With A Twist

Serves 6

Ingredients

1 packet elbow macaroni (16 oz.)
1 cup cooked parsnip, mashed
1 can haricot beans, drained and rinsed
1 cup kale, finely shredded
6 green onions, chopped

For the cashew cream
2 cups boiling water
1 cup raw cashews
Juice of one lemon
1 clove garlic, minced
1 teaspoon Dijon mustard
Cracked black pepper to taste
Pinch salt

To serve
3/4 cup toasted breadcrumbs

Method

1. Put the cashew nuts and boiling water into a bowl and set aside.

2. Meanwhile, cook the macaroni on your stove top in salted boiling water for around 10 minutes, or until al dente. Drain and reserve.
3. Now that the cashew nuts have soaked for around 10 minutes, put them into your food processor along with the other cashew cream ingredients. Blend to form a smooth paste.
4. Add the haricot beans and cooked parsnip to the food processor and pulse to combine. It's fine if the mix is now chunky.
5. Mix the contents of your food processor through the macaroni, along with the green onions and kale.
6. Coat the inside of your slow cooker with cooking spray and transfer the combined mixture to the slow cooker. Cook on low heat for 3 to 4 hours.
7. Toast the breadcrumbs in a skillet with a little olive oil and sprinkle over the dish when ready to serve.

Sweet Potato And Spinach Cannelloni

Serves 4 to 6

Ingredients

12 cannelloni shells, oven-ready
4 cups tomato sauce
1/4 cup vegan parmesan, shredded

For the stuffing
4 cups sweet potato, peeled, cooked and mashed
1 cup baby spinach, rinsed and chopped (if using frozen, defrost it)
1/2 cup almond meal (or breadcrumbs, if you prefer)
2 teaspoons dried oregano
Pinch salt
Pinch black pepper
Pinch ground nutmeg

Method

1. Grease your slow cooker with cooking spray.
2. Spread half of the tomato sauce on the bottom of the slow cooker.
3. In a large bowl, combine the spinach, sweet potato, almond meal and seasonings. If the mixture looks a little dry, add a splash of water.
4. Fill the cannelloni shells with the stuffing mixture.
5. Place these shells side by side in the slow cooker (you can make two layers if need be).

6. Pour the remaining sauce over the shells and sprinkle with the shredded parmesan.
7. Cook on high for 4 hours or on low for 6 to 8 hours.

Quinoa Pilaf

Serves 4

Ingredients

1 cup quinoa
1 celery stalk, finely chopped
1/2 red bell pepper, finely chopped
2 cups vegetable broth
2 tablespoons olive oil
1 teaspoon dried thyme
1 teaspoon smoked paprika
1 bay leaf
Pinch salt

To serve
1/2 cup almonds, roughly chopped
1/4 cup fresh parsley, roughly chopped
Freshly ground black pepper

Method

1. Add all the ingredients to your slow cooker and cook on low heat for 6 hours or on high for 3 hours.
2. Remove the bay leaf once the pilaf is cooked.
3. Before serving, heat a skillet on medium high heat and dry roast the almonds. Stir them through the pilaf, along with the chopped parsley, and grind some black pepper on top.

Pearl Barley With Broccoli And Spinach

Serves 4

Ingredients

1 1/2 cups pearl barley
1/2 head broccoli, cut into florets
1/2 packet frozen spinach (around 6 oz.)
2 1/2 cups vegetable stock
2 cups water
1 teaspoon dried thyme
Salt to taste

Method

1. Add all the ingredients to your slow cooker, mix well and cook on low heat for 4 to 6 hours, or until the barley is tender.
2. Serve as is, or sprinkle over some vegan parmesan, fresh parsley and cracked black pepper to make it extra special.

Mushroom And Pea Risotto

Serves 4

Ingredients

1 cup Arborio rice
1/2 cup button mushrooms, sliced
1 onion, chopped
2 garlic cloves, minced
2 tablespoons olive oil
1 cup frozen peas
1/2 cup dry white wine
3 cups vegetable stock, hot
1 tablespoon dried parsley
1/4 cup vegan parmesan, shredded

Method

1. Spray the inside of your slow cooker with cooking spray.
2. Heat the olive oil in a skillet and sauté the onion until softened.
3. Add the mushrooms, rice and garlic and sauté for another minute.
4. Place this mixture into your slow cooker. Add the wine, stock, peas and parsley and cook for 3 to 4 hours on low heat, or until the rice is tender.
5. Before serving, stir through the vegan parmesan and adjust the seasoning.

Stuff It!

Stuffed Tomatoes

Serves 4

Ingredients

4 tomatoes
1/2 cup silken tofu
1/2 cup almond meal
Handful black olives, pitted and chopped
1 teaspoon Dijon mustard
Handful fresh chives, chopped
Pinch salt

Method

1. Cut the tops off the tomatoes and scoop out the seeds and juicy pulp.
2. In a work bowl, mash the tofu with a fork, then mix through the almond meal, olives, mustard, chives and salt.
3. Stuff the mixture into the tomatoes and line them up in your slow cooker. Cook for 2 to 4 hours on low.

Stuffed Bell Peppers

Serves 6

Ingredients

6 bell peppers (any color)
1 can sweet corn
1 small onion, diced
1 can black beans, drained and rinsed
2 cups cooked long grain rice
1/2 teaspoon smoked paprika
1/4 teaspoon ground black pepper
1/4 teaspoon salt
1 cup tomato sauce
1/3 cup water

Method

1. Cut the top off the peppers and remove the membranes and seeds.
2. Combine the beans, onion, corn, rice and spices in a mixing bowl.
3. Stuff the bell peppers with this mix.
4. Carefully stand the bell peppers up in your slow cooker.
5. Pour the tomato sauce and water around the bell peppers.
6. Cook on high for 4 hours or on low for 6 to 7 hours.

Stuffed Zucchini Boats

Serves 4

Ingredients

2 large zucchinis
1/3 cup rice (raw)
1 1/2 cups tomato sauce
1 tablespoon balsamic vinegar
1 teaspoon dried basil
1 teaspoon garlic powder
Pinch salt and pepper

Method

1. Cut the zucchini in half lengthways. Use a spoon to scoop out the soft center. You should now have 4 zucchini boats. Lay your zucchini boats in the bottom of your slow cooker.
2. In a work bowl, combine the rice with the vinegar, basil, garlic powder, salt and pepper.
3. Spoon the raw rice mixture into your zucchini boats.
4. Pour the tomato sauce around the zucchini.
5. Cook on low for 6 to 8 hours, or until the rice is tender.

Cabbage Rolls

Serves 6

This recipe takes a little more effort but is great for stress-free entertaining. Simply prep everything in the morning and you can forget about it until you're ready to serve at night!

Ingredients

1 whole cabbage
4 green onions, finely shopped
1/2 cup white rice (raw)
1 can brown lentils, with juice
1 red bell pepper, finely diced
1 teaspoon dried basil
1 teaspoon dried oregano
1 teaspoon paprika
1 tablespoon onion powder
Pinch salt and pepper
2 cups tomato sauce

Method

1. Put a large pan of water on the stove and bring it to the boil (or boil the water in your electric jug to speed up the process).
2. Meanwhile, place the cabbage on your chopping board base side up and use a small paring knife to cut out the hard core.

3. Place the whole cabbage into the pan of boiling water. The cabbage leaves will start to soften and come away from the cabbage. Remember that you want the leaves whole! You can use a pair of tongs to gently pull the leaves away. You should aim to have 2 whole cabbage leaves for each person, so you'll need 12 leaves if you're serving 6 people. Reserve your cabbage leaves.
4. To make the stuffing, combine the rice, lentils (reserve the juice for later), bell pepper, onion and seasonings in a work bowl.
5. Lay a cabbage leaf flat and put a tablespoon of the stuffing mix into the center. Fold in the sides and then roll the cabbage up into a tight roll. Place the cabbage roll into the bottom of your slow cooker.
6. Repeat the above step until you have made 12 cabbage rolls.
7. Pour the tomato sauce and juice from the canned lentils over the top of the cabbage rolls.
8. Cook on low for 6 to 8 hours, or until the rice is tender.

Stews And Chili

Chinese Hot Pot

Serves 4 to 6

Ingredients

1 packet firm tofu (around 8 oz.), cubed
1 can baby corn
1 yellow onion, thinly sliced
1 carrot, thinly sliced
1 cup frozen peas
1 cup button mushrooms
2 tablespoons corn starch
3 cups vegetable stock
2 cloves garlic, minced
1 thumb ginger, minced
2 tablespoons soy sauce
1 teaspoon ground chili pepper (or more if you like spicy food)
1 tablespoon sesame seeds

Method

1. Whisk the cornstarch with 1/2 cup vegetable stock to form a paste. Once lump-free, place into the slow cooker and mix with the rest of the vegetable stock.
2. Place the remaining ingredients into your slow cooker and mix well to combine.

3. Cook on low for 4 to 6 hours.

Butternut Squash And Coconut Chili

Serves 6

Ingredients

1 medium onion, diced
1 carrot, diced
2 cups peeled and diced butternut squash
1 apple, peeled and diced
4 garlic cloves, finely minced (or 1 teaspoon garlic powder)
1 can garbanzo beans, drained and rinsed
1 can black beans, drained and rinsed
1 can coconut milk
2 cups vegetable broth
2 teaspoons ground cumin
2 teaspoons ground coriander
2 teaspoons ground chili pepper
2 tablespoons tomato concentrate

Method

1. Put all the ingredients into the slow cooker. The liquid should cover the butternut squash, so add a little water if you need more liquid.
2. Cook on low heat for 8 hours or on high heat for 4 to 6 hours.

3. Keep the lid of the cooker open for the last 45 minutes to let the chili thicken.
4. Adjust the seasoning if desired and serve with basmati rice and fresh cilantro.

Super Easy Black Beans

Serves 4 to 6

Ingredients

2 cans black beans, drained and rinsed
2 cups vegetable broth
1 yellow onion, diced
2 garlic cloves, minced
1 tablespoon ground chili pepper
1 teaspoon cumin seeds
1 teaspoon ground coriander

Method

1. Place all the ingredients into the slow cooker and stir them together.
2. Cook on low for 6 to 8 hours. Once cooked, add salt to taste if desired.
3. These black beans are delicious served on soft corn tortillas with diced avocado.

Portuguese Fava Beans

Serves 4

Ingredients

2 cans fava beans, drained and rinsed
1 yellow onion, diced
3 cloves garlic, minced
1 tablespoon paprika
1/2 red bell pepper, finely diced
1 tablespoon tomato concentrate
2 cups vegetable stock
1/2 teaspoon chili pepper flakes
1/2 teaspoon black pepper

To serve
Handful fresh parsley, roughly chopped

Method

1. Put all the ingredients (except the parsley) into the slow cooker and stir to combine.
2. Cook for 4 hours on high heat or for 6 on low.
3. Sprinkle over the fresh parsley and serve hot with rice or bread.

Easy Italian Lentils

Serves 4

Ingredients

2 cans brown lentils, drained and rinsed
1 cup tomato sauce
1 tablespoon tomato concentrate
1 tablespoon balsamic vinegar
2 tablespoons brown sugar
1 teaspoon onion powder
1 teaspoon garlic powder
1 teaspoon dried oregano
1 teaspoon dried basil
1/2 cup water

Method

1. Add all the above ingredients to your slow cooker and mix well.
2. Cook on low heat for 6 hours or on high heat for 3 hours.
3. Serve on slider buns with your favorite garnishes.

Creamy Sweet Potato Stew

Serves 6

Ingredients

6 medium sweet potatoes, peeled and sliced
2 red onions, thinly sliced
1 clove garlic, minced
1 can tomatoes, diced
1 1/2 teaspoons ground cumin

To serve
Handful chopped fresh parsley
1/2 cup peanut butter, crunchy or smooth

Method

1. Put all the ingredients (except the peanut butter and parsley) into the slow cooker and stir to combine. Add enough water so that the liquid sits just above the sweet potatoes.
2. Cook on high for 4 to 6 hours, or until the sweet potatoes are very tender.
3. Just before serving the stew, stir through the peanut butter and chopped parsley. Season to taste.

Classic Veggie Chili

Serves 8

Ingredients

1 can kidney beans, drained and rinsed
1 can pinto beans, drained and rinsed
1 can black beans, drained and rinsed
1 can sweet corn, drained and rinsed
1 can fire-roasted tomatoes, diced
1 cup tomato sauce
1 cup water
1 tablespoon olive oil
1 large yellow onion, diced
3 garlic cloves, minced
2 small jalapeno peppers, seeded and minced
1 green bell pepper, diced

Method

1. Heat the olive oil in a pan and sauté the onion, green bell pepper and jalapeno over medium heat until all the ingredients soften. Add the garlic and sauté for a further 30 seconds.
2. Transfer the mixture to the slow cooker, add all the other ingredients and combine well.
3. Cook on low for 6 to 8 hours.
4. Serve on sliders with your favorite toppings, or with rice.

Curries

Indian-Inspired Cauliflower And Garbanzo Bean Curry

Serves 6 to 8

Ingredients

1 medium head of cauliflower, cut into bite-sized florets
2 potatoes, diced
1 eggplant, diced
1 large onion, diced
2 cans garbanzo beans, drained and rinsed
1 can coconut milk
1 can tomatoes, diced with juices
2 cups vegetable broth
3 cloves garlic, minced
1 tablespoon grated ginger
1 tablespoon curry powder
1 tablespoon palm sugar
1 tablespoon vegetable oil
1 teaspoon ground turmeric
Pinch salt

Method

1. Heat the oil in a skillet over medium heat.

2. Sauté the onion until soft and translucent. Add the ginger, garlic, and spices and sauté for a further 30 seconds until fragrant.
3. Remove the skillet from the heat and add a little broth to deglaze.
4. Pour this mixture in the slow cooker.
5. Add all the other ingredients.
6. Stir well and ensure that the liquid covers the vegetables. If necessary, add a little water.
7. Cover and cook on high for 4 to 6 hours or on low for 8 to 10 hours.

Cashew Cream Veggie Korma

Serves 6 to 8

This dish takes a tiny bit more prep, so it's perfect for the weekend. It's also great for stress-free entertaining – I've wowed lots of guests with it!

Ingredients

2 cups whole button mushrooms
1/2 medium butternut squash, cubed
3 potatoes, cubed
2 cups green beans, trimmed
3 cups vegetable stock
1 cup raw cashews

For the curry paste
1 tablespoon oil (use vegetable, peanut or coconut oil - not olive oil)
1 thumb ginger, minced
3 cloves garlic, minced
1 1/2 teaspoons ground cumin
1 1/2 teaspoons ground coriander
1/2 teaspoon ground chili pepper (or more, if you prefer)
1/2 teaspoon ground cinnamon
1/2 teaspoon ground turmeric

Method

1. Place the cashews into a bowl of boiling water and leave them to soak for an hour. While you're waiting, you can prep the rest of the ingredients, otherwise you can come back once the cashews have softened and continue the recipe.
2. Drain the cashew nuts and put them in your food processer along with two cups of the vegetable stock. Process until it forms a smooth, creamy paste. Reserve.
3. Heat the oil in a skillet and add all of the curry paste ingredients. Sauté for around a minute, or until fragrant. Be careful not to burn the curry paste!
1.
4. Combine the cashew paste, curry paste and all the other ingredients in your slow cooker.
5. Cook for 6 hours on low or 3 hours on high. Season to taste and serve with rice or Indian roti bread.

Malaysian Laksa

Serves 4 to 6

Ingredients

1 red bell pepper, thinly sliced
1 carrot, thinly sliced
1 can coconut milk
3 cups vegetable stock
1 lemon grass stem (whole)
3 kaffir lime leaves (fresh or dried)
1 red chili pepper, thinly sliced
1 tablespoon tamari or soy sauce
1 teaspoon sesame oil
1 teaspoon ground turmeric
1 tablespoon palm sugar (or raw brown sugar)
Juice of one lime
1 tablespoon oil (use vegetable, peanut or coconut oil - not olive oil)
1 thumb ginger, minced
3 cloves garlic, minced

To serve
1 cup bean sprouts
1 pack silken tofu (around 8 oz.), diced
1 cup baby spinach leaves
4 green onions, thinly sliced
Handful fresh coriander, roughly chopped
1 pack rice vermicelli noodles (around 10 oz.)

Method

1. Heat the oil in a skillet and sauté the garlic and ginger for around a minute, or until fragrant.
2. Combine the sautéed garlic and ginger in your slow cooker along with all the other ingredients.
3. Cook on low for 3 to 4 hours.
4. Remove the lemongrass stalk and kaffir lime leaves and adjust the seasoning to taste.
5. Cook the rice vermicelli according to packet directions.
6. Add the rice vermicelli, bean sprouts, tofu, spinach, green onions and coriander to the slow cooker. Serve in bowls.

Alternatively, to serve this laksa at a dinner party, place the rice vermicelli into the bottom of individual bowls, ladle over the laksa, then top with the bean sprouts, tofu, spinach, green onions and coriander – your guests will love this gorgeous presentation and delicious Malaysian laksa!

Breads

Vegan Egg Replacer

It's handy to know what to use in cakes and other recipes which normally call for eggs. An easy vegan egg replacer can be made from ground flax seeds. For each egg replacer, simply grind 1 tablespoon of flax seed in your food processor until it's nice and fine. Then simply mix the ground flax meal with 3 tablespoons of water and let the mix sit for 5 to 10 minutes. You'll now have a sticky mix that's the perfect vegan egg replacer.

Healthy Banana And Walnut Loaf

Makes one loaf

Ingredients

2 cups all-purpose whole wheat flour (or gluten-free flour)
2 teaspoons baking powder
1/2 teaspoon ground cinnamon
1 vegan egg replacer (see recipe at the start of the bread chapter)
2 large ripe bananas, mashed
1/2 cup water
1/2 cup raw sugar
1/4 cup melted coconut oil
1/2 cup chopped walnuts

Method

1. Combine the dry ingredients in a large work bowl (flour, baking powder, sugar and cinnamon).
2. Combine the wet ingredients in another work bowl (mashed banana, egg replacer, coconut oil and water).
3. Mix the wet ingredients into the dry. Lastly, stir through the chopped walnuts.
4. Take a loaf pan that fits inside your slow cooker. Grease the pan with cooking spray or oil and pour the batter in.
5. Place the loaf pan inside the slow cooker. Cook on high for around 2 hours or until a toothpick inserted into the center comes out clean.

Corn Bread

Makes one loaf

Ingredients

3/4 cup cornmeal
1 cup all-purpose flour
2 teaspoons baking powder
1 cup sweet corn kernels (frozen is fine)
2 tablespoons sugar
3/4 cup coconut milk, unsweetened
1 vegan egg replacer (see recipe at the start of the bread chapter)
2 tablespoons vegetable oil
1 teaspoon salt

Method

1. Spray the inside of your slow cooker with cooking spray.
2. Combine the cornmeal, baking powder, sugar, salt and all-purpose flour in a bowl.
3. Combine the vegan egg replacer, oil, coconut milk and corn in a separate bowl.
4. Now combine the wet ingredients with the dry.
5. Pour the cornbread batter into your greased slow cooker. (Note: if you have a large slow cooker, you may prefer to use a loaf pan and place it inside the slow cooker. Of course, you can make a very thin,

flat cornbread slice directly in your large slow cooker.)
6. Cook on high heat for around 2 hours, or until a toothpick inserted into the cornbread comes out clean. Each slow cooker is different, so check after 1 1/2 hours, then keep checking at 1/2 hour intervals.

Rosemary Bread

Makes one loaf

Ingredients

3 cups all-purpose flour
1 tablespoon active dry yeast
1 1/4 cups warm water
Handful fresh rosemary, chopped
1 tablespoon sugar
1 tablespoon salt

Method

1. Mix the yeast, sugar and water in a bowl and set it aside for 10 minutes so that the yeast activates (the mixture should form bubbles). Note that the water should be body temperature – if it's too hot, you'll kill the yeast, too cold and it won't activate.
2. Combine the activated yeast mix with all the other ingredients until it forms a dough. Each brand of flour is different, so add a little more water if your dough is too dry.
3. Grease a large bowl and put the dough inside it.
4. Cover the bowl with plastic wrap and leave it in a draft-free, warm place for 1 hour so the dough can rise.
5. Flour your bench and knead the dough, folding it over itself and pushing it out again. Knead for

around 15 minutes, or until the dough becomes elastic.
6. Place the dough back into the bowl, cover and leave it to proof for a further half hour.
7. Put your slow cooker on high heat and line the bottom with a sheet of parchment paper.
8. Put the dough inside the slow cooker. Cover the dough with paper towel and then put the lid on (this will prevent the moisture from dripping back onto the top of the bread).
9. Cook for 2 hours on high. Cook time may vary depending on your specific slow cooker, so it's a good idea to check the bread after an hour. You know the bread's cooked when a knife inserted into the center comes out clean or the internal temperature reaches around 200 degrees Fahrenheit (90 degrees Celsius).
10. You can use this same recipe to make lots of different breads by simply swapping the rosemary with other ingredients. Some other delicious options include 1/2 cup chopped Kalamata olives 1/2 cup chopped sundried tomatoes or 1/2 cup chopped walnuts.

Desserts

Rice Pudding

Serves 6

Ingredients

1 cup short grain rice
2 cups coconut milk
1 cup water
1/2 brown sugar
1/2 cup raisins
1 cinnamon stick
1 teaspoon vanilla extract

Method

1. Spray the inside of your slow cooker with cooking spray.
2. Combine all the ingredients in your slow cooker. Cook on high for 2 to 3 hours or low for 4 to 6 hours, or until the rice is tender and creamy.
3. Remove the cinnamon stick before serving. Enjoy warm or chilled.

Cranberry And Peach Crumble

Serves 4

Ingredients

6 peaches, sliced
1/3 cup dried cranberries
1/2 cup quick cooking oats
1/2 cup brown sugar
4 tablespoons coconut oil, melted
2 tablespoons all-purpose flour
2 tablespoons flaked almonds
1/2 teaspoon ground cinnamon

Method

1. Place the peaches in the bottom of your slow cooker.
2. Combine the remaining ingredients in a bowl.
3. Sprinkle the crumble mixture over the peaches.
4. Cook on low heat for 4 hours or high for 2.

Pumpkin Pudding

Serves 6 to 8

Ingredients

2 cups all-purpose flour
1 cup cooked and mashed pumpkin
3 teaspoons baking powder
3/4 cup brown sugar
1 cup coconut cream
1 teaspoon vanilla extract
2 tablespoons coconut oil, melted
2 teaspoons pumpkin pie spice

Method

1. Grease your slow cooker with cooking spray.
2. Mix all the ingredients in a work bowl. Depending on how dry your pumpkin is, you may need to add a little water. You're aiming to form a very wet, loose dough or very stiff batter, depending on which way you like to think of it!
3. Transfer the mix to the slow cooker.
4. Cook on low heat for 6 hours or high for 2 to 3.

Stewed Rhubarb And Strawberry Sauce

Serves 4 to 6

Ingredients

1 cup strawberries, quartered
4 cups rhubarb, chopped
1/2 cup water
1 cup raw sugar
1 thumb ginger, minced
1 teaspoon ground cinnamon
Pinch ground cloves

Method

1. Spray the inside of your slow cooker with cooking spray.

2. Add all the ingredients to the slow cooker.

3. Cover and cook on high for 2 hours or low for 4.

4. Remove the mixture and blend until smooth.

5. Serve warm or chilled with soy yoghurt or soy ice-cream.

Chocolate Peanut Butter Cake

Makes one cake

Ingredients

For the cake
1 cup all-purpose flour
1/2 cup raw sugar
2 tablespoons coconut butter, melted
1 1/2 teaspoons baking powder
1/2 cup soy milk
1 teaspoon vanilla extract
3/4 cup chocolate chips
1/2 cup smooth peanut butter
1/2 cup boiling water

For the sauce
1/2 cup rice syrup (or any other vegan syrup)
4 tablespoons raw cocoa powder
1 cup boiling water

Method

1. Combine the peanut butter with 1/2 cup boiling water and mix until the paste is lump-free.
2. Mix through the vanilla extract, melted coconut butter and soy milk.
3. In a separate bowl, combine the flour, baking powder and sugar.

4. Mix the wet ingredients through the dry ingredients. Then add the choc chips.
5. Spoon the cake mix into your greased slow cooker.
6. Make the sauce by mixing together the rice syrup, cocoa powder and water.
7. Pour the sauce over the cake.
8. Cook on high for 2 1/2 hours.

Soups & Stews

Curried Vegetables And Chickpea Stew

This is a delicious stew that is simple to make and can be made with leftover vegetables and a can of chickpeas. It can be high in sodium however, so skip the salt if you wish.

Ingredients

1 teaspoon of olive oil
1 large diced onion
2 diced potatoes
1 tablespoon curry powder
1 tablespoon brown sugar
1 tablespoon salt
3 minced garlic cloves
1 inch piece of peeled and grated ginger
1 can diced of tomatoes with their juices
2 (16 ounce) cans of drained and rinsed chickpeas
1/8 teaspoon cayenne pepper
2 cups vegetable broth
1 diced green bell pepper
1 diced red bell pepper
1 cauliflower medium sized head cut into bite-sized florets
¼ teaspoon black pepper
10 ounces of baby spinach

1 cup coconut milk

Method

1. Into a skillet, heat the oil and add the onion, sautéing with the teaspoon of salt until it's then translucent, which should take about 5 minutes. Add in the potatoes along with a teaspoon of salt and sauté until the edges also become translucent.
2. Stir in the brown sugar, garlic, ginger, curry powder and the chili until the mixture becomes fragrant, which should take about 30 seconds. Pour in the ¼ cup of broth, making sure that you scrape the bottom of the pan to ensure it's deglazed.
3. Into the slow cooker, add the chickpeas, broth, cauliflower, bell pepper, tomatoes and their juices. Add in the pepper and the final teaspoon of salt. Make sure to stir well to combine all of the ingredients. The liquid should be halfway up to the sides of the bowl, and be sure to add in more broth if necessary.
4. Cover and then allow to cook in the slow cooker for 4 hours on a high heat. Stir in the spinach along with the coconut milk and cover the lid for 1 minute until the spinach starts to wilt. Taste and then adjust the salt as necessary, along with other seasonings. Serve with cous cous or on its own as desired.

Serves: 8-10

Calories (Total): 914kcal. Carbs: 146g 53%. Protein: 26g 24%, Fat: 25g 34%, Saturated Fat: 7.2g 29%, Cholesterol: 0mg, Sodium: 3,662 244%, Fiber: 26g 105%, Sugar: 35g 35%, Vitamin A: 2091IU, Vitamin C: 339mg, Calcium: 692mg 69%, Iron 9.1mg 51%, Potassium: 2,288 49%

Indian Spiced Lentils

These Indian spiced lentils make an excellent and comforting dish, especially when served with rice or quinoa.

Ingredients

2 cups of red lentils
10 ounces spinach
1 chopped onion
1 15 ounce can of diced tomatoes
1 tablespoon of minced garlic
1 tablespoon of minced fresh ginger
4 cups of vegetable broth
1 teaspoon mustard seeds
½ teaspoon ground cumin
1/8-1/4 teaspoon cayenne pepper
Juice of ½ a lemon or a lime
2 teaspoons sugar
1 ½ teaspoons kosher salt
1 teaspoon curry powder or paste
Handful of chopped cilantro

Method

1. Add all of the above ingredients into the slow cooker, except for the lemon or lime juice and the cilantro.

2. Cook on a high temperature for 3-4 hours, or for 6-7 hours on a low heat. Bring to the boil on the stove and then simmer while covered for 1 hour.
3. Before you serve the dish, add in the lemon juice and the cilantro. This is especially delicious when served with rice or quinoa, but you might want to consider naan bread or poppadoms instead.

Serves: 8

Calories (Total): 790kcal 36%. Carbs: 146g 53%. Protein: 49g 45%, Fat: 4.1g 6%, Saturated Fat: 0.5g 2%, Cholesterol: 0g 0%. Sodium: 3,539mg 236%. Fiber: 43g 172%. Sugar: 44g, 80%. Vitamin A: 29,484+ 590%. Vitamin C: 130mg 173%. Calcium: 532mg 53%. Iron: 26mg, 142%. Potassium: 3,277mg 70%.

'Cream' Of Mushroom Soup

This 'creamy' mushroom soup is a perfect winter warmer – without any added dairy.

Ingredients

2 tablespoons of extra virgin olive oil
1 diced yellow onion
2 diced garlic cloves
10 diced button mushrooms
6-8 sliced baby Portobello mushrooms
2 medium/large diced and peeled potatoes
¼ cup of white wine
4 cups of plain unsweetened soy milk
3 teaspoons of sweet white miso
Finely minced fresh parsley for garnishing

Method

1. In a large pot heat some oil and sauté the onions and garlic together for 2-3 minutes.
2. Stir in the mushrooms and the potatoes, sautéing for an extra 2-3 minutes.
3. Add the soy milk, wine, salt and pepper into the mixture. Cover and then bring to the boil. Reduce this heat to a low temperature and cook for one hour.

4. Once the soup has been heated, pour into a blender and blend until the mixture becomes creamy. Add back into the pot.
5. Add a small amount of the soup into a bowl and then stir in the miso, allowing it to dissolve. Cook over a low heat uncovered, for up to 3 to minutes.
6. Salt and pepper can be used for seasoning and fresh parsley can be used to garnish.

Serves: **4-5**

Calories (Total): 1534kcal (383.5kcal a serving). Carbs: 216g 79%. Protein: 60g 54%. Fat: 51g 6.9%. Cholesterol: 0mg 0%. Sodium: 639mg 43%. Fiber: 26g 103%. Sugar: 54g 99%. Vitamin A: 5,102IU 102%. Vitamin C: 150mg 201%. Calcium: 476mg 48%. Iron: 15.4g 86%. Potassium: 4,477mg 95%.

White Bean Soup

This hearty soup is ideal for keeping you warm during winter.

Ingredients

2 tablespoons of olive oil
4 garlic cloves
1 medium yellow onion
1/2lb carrots
1lb dry navy beans
4 celery stalks
1 whole bay leaf
1 tsp dried rosemary
½ tsp dried thyme
½ tsp smoked paprika
Freshly cracked pepper

Method

1. Mince the onion, garlic, celery and slice the carrots. Add the olive oil, onion, garlic, carrots and the celery into a large slow cooker.
2. Give the beans a rinse and add them into the slow cooker along with thyme, rosemary, bay leaf, paprika and freshly cracked pepper.
3. Into the slow cooker add six cups of water, stirring and combining the ingredients. Place the lid on the

top of the slow cooker and cook for 8 hours on a low setting.
4. After 8 hours, be sure to stir the soup and mash the beans a little. Add ½ a teaspoon of salt in as you desire. Ladle into bowls and serve with bread.

Serves: 6-8

Calories (Total): 708kcal 32%. Carbs: 92g 34%. Protein: 24g 22%. Fat: 30g 40%. Saturated Fat: 4.4g 18%. Cholesterol: 0mg. Sodium: 4,818mg 321%. Fiber: 25g 99%. Sugar: 24g 44%. Vitamin A: 768IU 15%. Vitamin C:80mg 106%. Calcium: 229mg 23%. Iron: 6.4mg 36%. Potassium: 2,532mg 54%.

Chickpea, Butternut Squash And Red Lentil Stew

This tasty stew is an exciting way to use butternut squash and red lentils together to create a meal that's both colorful and delicious.

Ingredients

1 chopped yellow onion
1 chopped large carrot
2 cloves of minced garlic
1 butternut squash, peeled and chopped
1 seeded and minced jalapeno
2-3 tsp garam masala
1 28oz can diced tomatoes in tomato juice
1 cup red lentils
2 15oz cans of drained and rinsed chickpeas
1-2 tsp sea salt
1 quart vegetable broth
1 tbsp olive or canola oil
Freshly minced cilantro for serving

Method

1. Into a large skillet add the oil over a medium high heat. Add in the carrot, onion and jalapeno, sautéing for six minutes. Add in the minced garlic for another 30 seconds and then add in the garam

masala, stirring in the mixture and coating it well. Remove from the heat.
2. Place the onion mixture, butternut squash, chickpeas, red lentils, canned diced tomatoes and the vegetable broth into your slow cooker. Turn the heat on low and cook for an average of 8-10 hours. The longer this is cooked, the thicker the stew will be.
3. Add seasoning with sea salt to taste and then serve with the minced cilantro on top of the dish. This stew will freeze well and can be kept in the fridge for 5 days.

Serves: 4-6

Calories (Total): 1142kcal 115%. Carbs: 421g 153%. Protein: 138g 125%. Fat: 40g 55%. Saturated Fat: 40g 55%. Cholesterol: 0mg 0%. Sodium: 6,167mg 411%. Fiber: 110g 441%. Sugar: 83g 151%. Vitamin A: 5,649IU 113%. Vitamin C: 662mg 66%. Iron:47mg 261%. Potassium: 5,087mg 108%.

Crockpot Thai Coconut Soup

An exciting Asian soup that's full of spice and flavor, this recipe is easy to prepare and is excellent as a starter or on its own.

Ingredients
8oz extra firm tofu cut into small cubes
3 tbsp thai curry paste
1 tbsp canola oil
6 thai basil leaves (torn)
2 tsp brown sugar
½ tsp salt
1 14oz can coconut milk
2 cups vegetable broth
1 6-inch stalk lemongrass
½ a lime, juiced
2 red or green Thai chillies
½ cup dry jasmine rice
Cilantro (for garnishing)

Method

1. In a cup, cook the rice using a half a cup of water until the rice is tender. This should take about 30 minutes. Fluff the rice and then place aside.
2. Use a teaspoon of oil to heat a large nonstick skillet on a high heat. Add in the cubed tofu, curry paste, mashing them together in the oil until the mixture is well combined. Stir as you cook for another 2

minutes and then whisk it in slowly with the broth and the coconut milk.
3. After adding in the vegetable broth, add the brown sugar, salt, Thai basil, lemongrass stalk, lime juice and chilies, stirring for ten minutes. Place in the slow cooker and allow the flavors to develop for 1-2 hours.
4. Add in the cooked rice to individual bowls (or place in the slow cooker first with the liquid, depending on your preferences). Ladle the soup in and sprinkle with the chopped cilantro. Before serving the soup, remember to remove the chilies and lemongrass (you don't want to eat these).

Serves: 4

Calories (Total): 956kcal 43%. Carbs: 104g 38%. Protein: 25g 22%. Fat: 46g 63%. Fat: 46g 63%. Saturated Fat: 23g 95%. Cholesterol: 0mg 0%. Sodium: 3,103mg 207%. Fiber: 2g 8%. Sugar: 16.6g 30%. Vitamin A: 7,750IU 155%. Vitamin C: 4.1mg 5%. Calcium: 516mg 52%. Iron: 7.7mg, 43%. Potassium: 335mg 7%.

Potato Zucchini Soup

This soup will keep you feeling full and is an excellent idea for a meal when you're feeling lazy.

Ingredients

9 cups vegetable broth
6 cups of peeled, diced potatoes
1 large zucchini, quartered and thinly sliced
1 large sweet onion
3 cloves of garlic
1 tbsp extra virgin olive oil
½ tsp curry powder (optional)
Sea salt (to taste)
Freshly grated pepper (to taste)

Method

1. Add the vegetable broth into the large slow cooker. Peel and then dice the potatoes, adding those in.
2. Into a large skillet, add olive oil and heat to a medium-high temperature. As the skillet is heating up, chop the onions and quarter the zucchini, slicing thinly. Add this to the skillet, stirring occasionally.
3. Halfway through the cooking, add some garlic and then when the onions and zucchini are starting to become translucent, transfer this into the slow cooker.

4. Stir in the sea salt, pepper and curry powder. Allow to slow cook for 6-8 hours on a low temperature. In the last half hour of cooking, use the immersion blender for 15 seconds in one area. Stir this and then check for the appearance and taste.
2. For a thicker soup, repeat with the immersion blender. Cook for an extra 30 minutes. Serve the soup with some lovely gluten free bread.

Serves: **4**

Calories (Total): 1112kcal 51%. Carbohydrates: 226g, 82%. Protein: 18.9g, 17%. Fat: 15g 20%. Saturated Fat: 2.2g 9%. Cholesterol: 0mg 0%. Sodium: 8,603mg 574%. Fiber: 19.1g 76%. Sugar: 34g 61%. Vitamin A: 4,606IU, 92%. Vitamin C: 133mg, 178%. Calcium: 70mg 7%. Iron: 3mg 17%. Potassium: 3,791mg 81%.

Butternut Squash And Parsnip Soup

This soup is a perfect winter warmer and is also high in Vitamin A and potassium.

Ingredients

2 large parsnips, peeled and chopped
1 large yellow onion, chopped
1 fuji apple, peeled and chopped
1 small butternut squash, peeled, seeds and chopped into small squares (about 5 cups)
2 cups low sodium vegetable broth
1/8 teaspoon ground sage
½ teaspoon ground cumin
¼ teaspoon dried thyme
½ teaspoon ground coriander
½ teaspoon salt

Method:

1. Add all of the above ingredients into a crock pot and cook on a low temperature for 6 hours.
2. After the vegetables are cooked, add the soup to a blender and blend the mixture until smooth.

Serves: 4-6 people
Calories (Total): 585kcal 27%. Carbohydrates: 144g 52%. Protein: 9g 8%. Fat: 0.7g 1%. Saturated Fat: 0.2g

1%. Cholesterol: 0mg 0%. Sodium: 328mg 22%. Fiber: 29g 116%. Sugar: 44g 81%. Vitamin A: 74,510+ 1490+. Vitamin C: 195mg 44%. Calcium: 436mg 44%. Iron: 6.7mg 37%. Potassium: 3,224mg 69%.

African Peanut Stew

This tasty African stew is high in Vitamin A and a good source of carbohydrates and protein, meaning it will keep you feeling fuller for longer.

Ingredients

2 medium sized sweet potatoes, peeled and then chopped into bite-sized pieces
1 large sweet onion, chopped
1 large red bell pepper, or 2 small ones, chopped
2 heaped tablespoons peanut butter
¼ cup dark brown sugar
¾ teaspoon salt
1 (14.5 ounce) can lite coconut milk
1 (15-19 ounces) can garbanzo beans, rinsed and drained
1 14.5 ounce can of diced tomatoes
2 inches of fresh ginger, peeled
1 teaspoon ground cumin
½ teaspoon ground cinnamon
¼ teaspoon ground red pepper (cayenne)
1 tablespoon curry powder
3-4 garlic cloves

1 cup loosely packed fresh cilantro leaves and stems

Method:
1. Into a food processor add the garlic cloves, cilantro, ginger, tomatoes, cumin, cinnamon, peanut butter, curry powder and ground red pepper. Blend this until the mixture is pureed and looks thick and pasty.
2. Into the slow cooker add the chopped onions, red bell peppers, garbanzo beans and the sweet potatoes. Add in the brown sugar, coconut milk, peanut sauce mixture, stirring to gently mix all of the ingredients together.
3. Turn the slow cooker on to a low temperature and then cook for 6-8 hours. Serve the stew with rice and top with some sliced green onions and fresh cilantro.

Serves: **4-6**
Calories (Total): 1525kcal 69%. Carbohydrates: 266g 97%. Protein: 45g 41%. Fat: 43g 58%. Saturated Fat: 23g 92%. Cholesterol: 0mg 0%. Sodium: 2,495mg 166%. Fiber: 42g 168%. Sugar: 99g 180%. Vitamin A: 45,803+ 916%. Vitamin C: 297mg 396%. Calcium: 377mg 38%. Iron: 15.6mg 87%. Potassium: 2,256mg 48%.

Hearty Vegetable And Bean Soup

The ideal soup to make on a rainy day, curled up on the sofa and watching the world pass by. This healthy soup is rich in protein, Vitamin A, iron and potassium.

Ingredients

2 cloves minced garlic
1 sweet onion, diced
1 medium sweet potato, peeled and cut into 1" cubes
2 celery stalks, diced
2 carrots, peeled and sliced into 1" pieces
1 cup whole kernel corn
1 bay leaf
1 teaspoon paprika
1/8 teaspoon allspice
½ teaspoon black pepper
Kosher or sea salt (to taste)
½ teaspoon crushed red pepper flakes
4 cups low sodium vegetable broth
2 cups fresh or frozen green beans
1 (14.5 oz) can diced tomatoes
2 cans cannellini beans, drained and rinsed

Method:

1. Place all of the above ingredients into a slow cooker, stirring to ensure they are thoroughly

combined. Cover and then cook for 8-10 hours on a low temperature, until the carrots become tender.
2. Serve with warm crusty bread and enjoy!

Serves: 6
Calories: (Total) 880kcal 40%. Carbohydrates: 180g 65%. Protein: 23g 21%. Fat: 3g 4%. Saturated Fat: 0.2g 1%. Cholesterol: 0.2mg 0%. Sodium: 2,583mg 172%. Fiber: 50g 200%. Sugar: 89g 143%. Vitamin A: 50,425+IU. Vitamin C: 193mg 257%. Calcium: 413mg 41%. Iron: 13.2mg 72%. Potassium: 3,813mg 81%.

Main Courses

Lentil Chili

A simple yet comforting dish that's perfect for any weather.

Ingredients

1 tablespoon of olive oil
2 medium chopped onions
6-8 minced garlic cloves
2 chopped carrots
1 chopped celery stalk
2 tablespoons chili powder
2 teaspoons cumin powder
1 teaspoon coriander powder
1 teaspoon dry mustard

1 teaspoon dried oregano
One 28 ounce box of crushed tomatoes
One 16 ounce package dry lentils
6-7 cups of vegetable broth
Salt to taste

Method

1. Into a large pot, heat some oil. Add in the garlic, onions, celery and carrot. Sauté the onions until they are lightly browned and soft, which should take about 3-4 minutes.
2. Add in the cumin, chili powder, oregano, coriander and mustard, stirring well for 1-2 minutes. Add in the tomatoes plus the salt to taste. Pour this mixture into the crockpot and then add in the lentils and the 6 cups of vegetable broth.
3. Cook for 4-6 hours, adding more water in as needed so you can achieve the desired consistency.

Serves: 12
Calories: (Total) 1222kcal 152%. Carbohydrates: 620g 225%. Protein: 109g 99%. Fat: 21g 29%. Saturated Fat: 2.9g 12%. Cholesterol: 0mg 0%. Sodium: 80,135+IU 5342%. Fiber: 139g 410%. Sugar: 226g 410%. Vitamin A: 44,867+IU 897%. Vitamin C: 125mg 167%. Calcium: 328mg 33%. Iron: 50mg 280%. Potassium: 1,004mg 21%.

Quinoa Jambalaya With Tempeh

This Caribbean dish takes some preparation, but is well worth it after a long day at the office. You can swap the vegetable bouillon for vegan based 'Not Chick'n' or 'Not Beef' bouillons instead for a more authentic flavor.

Ingredients

1 ½ cup of chopped bell pepper
3 minced garlic cloves
8 ounces of tempeh, cut into bite-sized pieces
1 ½ cups of diced tomatoes
1 teaspoon of vegetable bouillon
1-2 teaspoons Cajun seasoning
¼ to ½ teaspoon of liquid smoke or smoked paprika
3 cups water
¾ cup of quinoa, rinsed well
Tabasco sauce or hot pepper (optional)
Salt and pepper (to taste)

Method:

1. The night before you prepare this dish, place the tempeh and the vegetables in the fridge.
2. In the morning, add the chopped bell pepper, garlic cloves, tempeh, diced tomatoes, vegetable bouillon, Cajun seasoning, smoked paprika and the water into

the oiled slow cooker. Cook these ingredients on a low heat for 6-19 hours.
3. Around 1-2 hours before serving, ensure that the slow cooker is turned on high and add in the quinoa. Cook this until the quinoa starts to form white rings – that's when they're ready. Taste to ensure you are satisfied and then add in the Tabasco sauce, cayenne pepper and the salt if desired.

Serves: 4
Calories: (Total): 1072kcal 49%. Carbohydrates: 138g 50%. Protein: 64g 58%. Fat: 32g 43%. Saturated Fat: 5g 20%. Cholesterol: 0mg 0%. Sodium: 1047mg 70%. Fiber: 35g 138%. Sugar: 14.3g 26%. Vitamin A: 1624IU 32%. Vitamin C: 315mg 420%. Calcium: 280mg 28%. Iron: 15.3mg 85%. Potassium: 1597mg 34%.

Slow Cooker Chili

This delicious chili is easy to prepare and can then be left in the slow cooker for hours while you go about your day.

Ingredients

1 diced onion
1 red or yellow bell pepper (chopped)
2 carrots (grated or thinly sliced)
1 zucchini (diced)

2 cloves of minced garlic
2 cans of kidney beans
1 ½ cup corn
1 ½ tbsp chili powder
1 tsp cumin
2 15 ounce cans diced tomatoes
½ tsp red pepper flakes
A dash of cayenne pepper
A dash of Tabasco sauce (optional)

Method:

1. Take all of the above ingredients and place them into the slow cooker.
2. Cover the slow cooker and cook on a low heat for an average of 6-8 hours.

Serves: 5
Calories: (Total) 887kcal 40%. Carbohydrates: 171g 62%. Protein: 46g 42%. Fat: 5.2g 7%. Saturated Fat: 1.1g 5%. Cholesterol: 0mg 0%. Sodium: 2,537mg 169%. Fiber: 48g 193%. Sugar: 47g 86%. Vitamin A: 3,950IU 79%. Vitamin C: 378mg 505%. Calcium: 351mg 35%. Iron: 17.7mg 98%. Potassium: 4,506mg 96%.

Root Veggie Barley Risotto

A colorful and nutritious meal, the root veggies are an excellent source of vitamins and minerals.

Ingredients

2 cups (475ml) of water
½ cup of diced carrots
½ cup diced turnips or peeled rutabagas
½ cup (67g) of diced sweet potatoes or winter squash
2 minced garlic cloves
½ teaspoon dried oregano
½ teaspoon dried sage

1 cup (56g) minced greens like turnips, collards, kale, etc
½ teaspoon lemon zest
Salt and pepper (to taste

Method:

1. Add in all of the ingredients up to the minced greens, into the slow cooker. Cook on a low heat for 7-9 hours.
2. Around 30 minutes before the meal has to be served, add in the minced greens and the lemon zest. Add salt and pepper to taste just before serving and feel free to add in more sage and oregano if necessary.

Serves: 3

Calories (Total): 188 calories 9%. Carbohydrates: 42g 15%. Protein: 4.7g 4%. Fat: 1.1g 2% Saturated Fat: 0.4g 2%. Cholesterol: 0mg 0% Sodium: 650mg 43% Dietary Fiber: 10.2mg 41% Sugar: 18.4g 33% Vitamin A: 20,296+IU, 406% Vitamin C: 72mg 96% Calcium: 80mg 8% Iron: 3mg 17% Potassium: 1154mg 25%.

Crock Pot Bbq 'Beef'

Just because you're vegan doesn't mean you have to miss out on BBQ! This tasty alternative will please even the pickiest of meat eaters.

Ingredients

8oz fresh seitan
½ batch Homemade BBQ sauce (see ingredients below for how to prepare) or 1 bottle barbeque sauce
1 teaspoon garlic powder
1 teaspoon onion powder
Salt and pepper to taste
Wholemeal buns to serve (optional)
Salad to serve (optional)

Method:

1. Place the seitan, garlic and onion powder into the slow cooker, seasoning with salt and pepper.

2. Pour the barbeque sauce over the seitan. This should be cooked for 5-6 hours on a low temperature.
3. Remove the seitan from the slow cooker, shred and then return to the slow cooker for another 30 mins to 1 hour.

Homemade Bbq Sauce

Makes 2 cups

1 tbsp olive oil
2 cups ketchup
½ cup molasses
¼ cup diced white onion
2 tsp apple cider vinegar
1 tbsp liquid smoke
¼ cup vegan Worcestershire sauce
A pinch of cayenne

Method:
1. Heat oil in a medium sized pan. Add in the diced onions and sauté until the mixture becomes translucent. Let this cool. In the meantime add all the ingredients into a food processor or a blender, pureeing until smooth. Store this mixture in the refrigerator.

Serves: **8**

Calories: (Total): 835kcal 38%. Carbohydrates: 118g 43%. Protein: 53g 48%. Fat: 19g 26%. Saturated Fat: 2g 8%. Cholesterol: 0mg 0%. Sodium: 2,792mg 186%. Fiber: 2.8mg 11%. Sugar: 95g 172%. Vitamin A: 0IU 0%. Vitamin C: 2mg 3%. Calcium: 745mg 74%. Iron: 17.6mg 98%. Potassium: 1,994mg 42%.

Crock Pot Quinoa With Vegetables

Quinoa is an excellent source of proteins and essential amino acids. When combined with fresh green beans, carrots and sweet peppers it makes a delicious and highly nutritious meal.

Ingredients

1 small onion, chopped
1 tablespoon of olive oil
1 medium sweet red pepper, chopped
1 small carrot, chopped
1 cup fresh green beans, chopped
2 garlic cloves, minced
1 ½ cups quinoa
3 cups vegetable stock
1 teaspoon fresh cilantro or basil
¼ teaspoon black pepper

Method:

1. Rinse the quinoa thoroughly and then place it in the crock pot. Add the tablespoon of olive oil to coat the quinoa.
2. Stir in the vegetable broth, pepper, garlic and vegetables. Reserve the cilantro for later.
3. Cover the crock pot and cook for 4-6 hours on a low heat, or for 2-4 hours on a high heat.
4. Once the quinoa is done, fluff it using a fork and it should be tender. All of the liquid will have been absorbed into the quinoa.
3. Top the quinoa with fresh cilantro before serving.
4. Mix in the garbanzo or black beans to this dish. Serve and enjoy!

Serves: **4**

Calories: (Total): 1264kcal 57%. Carbohydrates: 210g 76%. Protein: 42g 38%. Fat: 30g 41%. Saturated Fat: 3.9g 16%. Cholesterol: 0mg 0%. Sodium: 3,024mg 202%. Fiber: 29mg 49%. Sugar: 27g 49%. Vitamin A: 6142IU 123%. Vitamin C: 193mg 257%. Calcium: 223mg 22%. Iron: 13.7mg 76%. Potassium: 2,149mg 46%.

Vegan Crock Pot Tacos

These crock pot tacos are delicious alternatives on a Mexican favorite. Enjoy!

Ingredients

1 onion, minced
1 tsp chili powder
1 tsp garlic powder
2 tsp cumin powder
1 tsp oregano
12 taco shells
2 cans (15oz) black beans
8oz can chopped green chilies
Your favorite toppings (e.g. tomatoes, jalapenos, vegan cheese, etc)

Method
1. Use a little nonstick spray in the slow cooker. Add all of the above ingredients, mixing well.
2. Cook on a low temperature for 6-8 hours, or a high of 3-5 hours.
3. Once the beans are cooked to the desired level, divide them between the eight taco shells.
4. Top with your favorite toppings and serve!

Serves: **6**

Calories: (Total): 838kcal 38%. Carbohydrates: 151g 55%. Protein: 32g 29%. Fat: 20g 28%. Saturated Fat: 4g 16%. Cholesterol: 0mg 0%. Sodium: 2,939mg 196%. Fiber: 28mg 112%. Sugar: 17.8g 32%. Vitamin A: 726IU 15%. Vitamin C: 23mg 31%. Calcium: 333mg 33%. Iron: 10.8mg 60%. Potassium: 1630mg 35%.

Vegan Brown Rice Mexican Bowl

A filling bowl of brown rice is a good source of protein and magnesium. It's made all the tastier with the beans, fresh vegetables and chilies for an extra spicy kick.

Ingredients

1 cup of long grain brown rice
2 cups of vegetable stock
1 cup finely chopped onion
1 red bell pepper
1 green bell pepper
4 ozs green chilies
15 ozs black beans
½ cup diced tomato
1 poblano pepper
½ a cup of thinly sliced green onion
½ cup freshly chopped cilantro
1 avocado
3 tbsps fresh lime juice
2 tbsps extra virgin olive oil
½ tsp ground cumin
Salt (to taste)

Method:

1. Place the rice, vegetable stock and the chopped onion into the slow cooker for one and a half hours until the rice is tenderized. As the rice is cooking, chop the red bell pepper and green pepper, opening

the diced green chilies. Drain the black beans into a colander in the sink and rinse with the cold water until no foam appears. Allow the beans to drain.
2. After an hour and a half, add in the red bell pepper, green peppers and chilies with the juice. Add in the drained black beans to the slow cooker and combine with the rice. Add salt for taste and allow to cook for 30 minutes on a high temperature.
3. When the rice mixture has finished cooking, chop in the tomato, cilantro and the thinly sliced green onion, along with the poblano pepper. Cut the avocado into 1 inch cubes across and toss this into a bowl with the fresh lime juice. Use the bowl to store all of the salsa ingredients. Make sure to add in the tomato, chopped cilantro, poblano, cumin, green onion, 3 tablespoons of lime juice, salt and the olive oil, combining to taste.
4. When the rice is tender, that is when the slow cooker mixture is ready. The vegan brown rice Mexican bowl can be served either hot or cold and is particularly delicious with homemade salsa.

Serves: 6
Calories (Total): 1,699kcal 77%. Carbohydrates: 256g 93%. Protein: 45g 41%. Fat: 64g 87%. Saturated Fat: 13g 53%. Cholesterol: 0mg 0%. Sodium: 3211mg 214%. Fiber: 63mg 250%. Sugar: 28g 51%. Vitamin A: 1911IU 38%. Vitamin C: 351mg 468%. Calcium: 183mg 18%. Iron: 12.5mg 69%. Potassium: 3211mg 68%.

Vegan Crock Pot Polenta Lasagna

This recipe is high in carbohydrates and protein, essential for fueling the body. It is also low in cholesterol, making it a healthier alternative to its meat equivalent.

Ingredients

Polenta:
1 cup polenta
1 tbsp margarine
4 cups water

Method:

1. Take a baking sheet and cover with parchment paper. Set it aside and bring 4 cups of water to the boil. Slowly add in the polenta. Add margarine, stirring until it's of a thick consistency.
2. Pour the polenta onto the prepared baking sheet, spreading evenly so it's ¼ inch thick. Set this aside to cool. Once this is cool, cut the polenta into rectangles.

Lasagna:
A dash of olive oil
½ bunch of kale, washed and chopped
1 large Portobello mushroom, cut into 1 inch slices
4 cloves of minced garlic

½ large onion, finely chopped
1 tsp dried basil
1-2 cups marinara sauce
'Cheese' sauce
Sea salt and pepper

Method:

1. Heat 1-2 tbsps of olive oil into a large skillet over a medium heat. Add in the onions and mushrooms, sautéing until juicy. Add the garlic in and cook for another 1-2 minutes.
2. Add the kale, cooking until it's a bright green color and soft. Add the 'cheese' sauce in and cook until this has thickened and is no longer runny. Remove this from the heat, seasoning with salt and pepper if desired.
3. Use the marinara sauce to coat the bottom of the crockpot. Cover with the marinara sauce and a single layer of polenta slices. Place the kale mixture on top and repeat this in layers: marinara sauce, polenta, kale; then finish with another layer of polenta then marinara.
4. Cover the crockpot and cook on a high temperature for 3-4 hours. Uncover this and leave to set aside for 30 minutes before serving onto plates.

'Cheese' Sauce

Ingredients

1/3 cup raw cashews
¼ cup nutritional yeast
1 cup unsweetened non-dairy milk
1 tbsp lemon juice
2 tsp Dijon mustard
½ tsp onion powder
½ tsp garlic powder
2 tsp corn starch or arrowroot
½ tsp white pepper

1. Place all of the above ingredients into a blender and pulse blend until smooth.

Serves: 2- 3
Calories (Total): 1092kcal 50%. Carbohydrates: 175g 64%. Protein: 27g 24%. Fat: 33g 44%. Saturated Fat: 7.6g 31%. Cholesterol: 0mg 0%. Sodium: 2,565mg 171%. Fiber: 15.9g 64%. Sugar: 24g 44%. Vitamin A: 20,438+IU 409%. Vitamin C: 68mg 90%. Calcium: 644mg 64%. Iron: 5.1mg 28%. Potassium: 430mg 9%.

Slow Cooker Spaghetti

A simple and 'skinny' alternative to traditional spaghetti Bolognese. Feel free to use meat-free vegan mince if necessary.

Ingredients

1 tablespoon extra virgin olive oil
1 small sweet onion, diced
2 cloves minced garlic
3 teaspoons capers, drained
2 teaspoons dried oregano
¼ teaspoon red pepper flakes
½ teaspoon black pepper
2 (14.5 ounce) cans fire roasted tomatoes
8 ounces whole wheat spaghetti, broken into small pieces
1 cup arugula

Method:

1. Add the oil into a small skillet and sauté the onion over a medium-low heat until tender which will take about 4 minutes.
2. Add in the garlic and sauté for an extra minute. Into a large bowl combine the sautéed onion and the garlic, along with the remaining ingredients, except for the arugula.
3. Toss all of the ingredients well and ensure that the spaghetti is coated with sauce, before adding into the slow cooker.
4. Cover the slow cooker and then place on a low heat for 2-3 hours until the pasta is al dente. Add in the arugula for the last 10 minutes of cooking, stirring to ensure it's well combined.
5. Serve onto a platter and sprinkle with vegan cheese if desired.

Serves: 4

Calories (Total): 565kcal 26%. Carbohydrates: 95g 35%. Protein:17.9mg 16%. Fat: 15.5g 21%. Saturated Fat: 2.3g 9%. Cholesterol: 0mg 0% Sodium: 1,797mg 120%. Fiber: 21g 85%. Sugar: 25g 46%. Vitamin A:2,268IU 45%. Vitamin C:48mg 64%. Calcium: 186mg 19% Iron: 5mg 28%. Potassium:184mg 4%.

Side Dishes

Slow Cooker Potatoes With Garlic And Rosemary

A 5-7 quart slow cooker is recommended for this particular recipe.

Ingredients

¼ cup extra virgin olive oil
3 cloves minced garlic
1 tablespoon chopped fresh rosemary
4 medium sized red potatoes, cubed into ½" pieces
½ teaspoon black pepper
Kosher or sea salt to taste

Method:

1. Into the slow cooker, add oil and turn to a high heat as you prepare the potatoes. Around 15 minutes of preheating is good.
2. Combine all of the above ingredients into the slow cooker, tossing the potatoes with oil, and then covering and cooking on a high heat for 2-3 hours (4-5 hours on low) until the potatoes become brown and tender.

Serves: 6

Calories (Total): 736kcal. Carbohydrates: 136g 49%. Protein: 15.9g 14%. Fat: 15g 20%. Saturated Fat: 2.2g 9%. Cholesterol: 0mg 0%. Sodium: 188mg 13%. Fiber: 12.5g 50%. Sugar: 9.9g 18%. Vitamin A: 69iu 1%. Vitamin C: 87mg 116%. Calcium: 62mg 6%. Iron: 4.8mg 27%. Potassium: 3,771mg 80%.

Slow Cooked Apples and Butternut Squash

A colorful side dish you can make in the slow cooker, perfect as an accompaniment to a roast dinner or Mediterranean dishes.

Ingredients

2-15oz cans fried apples
12 oz diced butternut squash

Method:
1. Use some cooking oil spray inside the slow cooker.
2. Place the butternut squash and the fried apples into the slow cooker and stir.
3. Cook on a low setting for 4 hours.

Serves: 6

Calories (Total): 1294kcal. Carbohydrates: 319g 116%. Protein: 3g 3%. Fat: 0.3g 0%. Saturated Fat: 0g 0%. Cholesterol: 0mg 0%. Sodium: 78mg 5%. Fiber: 24g 95%. Sugar: 257g 468%. Vitamin A: 758IU 15%. Vitamin C: 86mg 115%. Calcium: 13.3mg 1%. Iron: 11.6mg 64%. Potassium: 966mg 21%.

Slow Cooked Collard Greens

This is a good way to get greens into your diet. Collard greens are high in Vitamins A and C.

Ingredients

4 large bunches of collard greens (8 cups)
1 medium peeled white onion, diced
1 tablespoon raw apple cider vinegar
2 teaspoons coconut sugar
1 tablespoon extra virgin olive oil
4 peeled garlic cloves, minced
1 small dried chipotle chili pepper with the seeds and stems removed/diced
4 cups vegetable stock
2 tablespoons white wine

Method:
6. Prepare the collards for cooking. Remove the large ribs from the greens and stack the 4 or 5 leaves on top of one another, rolling them into a tight

cylinder. Slice them lengthwise into large ribbons. Make sure to place the cut greens into a clean and sterilized sink that's filled with cold water, along with 1 teaspoon of sea salt, cleaning them thoroughly. This can take a few changes of water to clean thoroughly.
7. Transfer the greens into a strainer or a salad spinner, allowing them to drain free of water.
8. Heat a tablespoon of olive oil into the large pot, over a medium heat. Add in the chipotle pepper, onions and the minced garlic. Cook this for 2 minutes, stirring it frequently so that all of the vegetables don't burn.
9. Add in the green collards, sprinkling them with apple cider vinegar along with a sweetener of your choice, black pepper and sea salt to taste.
10. Add in the vegetable stock and the wine to the slow cooker, covering and cooking for 45-60 minutes until the vegetables become tender. Taste and then adjust the seasoning if desired.

Serves: 4-6

Calories (Total): 662kcal 30%. Carbohydrates: 104g 38%. Protein: 33g 30%. Fat: 19.5g 27%. Saturated Fat: 2.7g 11%. Cholesterol: 0mg 0%. Sodium: 7732mg 515%. Fiber: 44g 174%. Sugar: 26g 46%. Vitamin A: 102,000+IU 2040%. Vitamin C: 283mg 377%. Calcium: 2150mg 215%. Iron: 17.7mg 98%. Potassium: 1800mg 38%.

Slow-Cooked Baked Beans

Slow cooked baked beans develop a distinct flavor and make the perfect side dish to any veggie burger.

Ingredients

1 medium yellow onion, diced
1 pound dried navy or pea beans
2½ cups water, plus more for soaking the beans
½ cup ketchup
¼ cup packed dark brown sugar
1 tablespoon Dijon mustard
¼ cup dark molasses
1 tablespoon kosher salt
1/8 teaspoon ground cloves
½ teaspoon freshly ground black pepper

Method:

1. Into a large bowl place the beans and pick through them, discarding any beans or stones as necessary. Cover the beans with at least 3 inches of cold water and allow to soak uncovered at a room temperature for about 8 hours overnight.
2. Drain in a colander and then reserve the bowl, setting it aside. Place the beans and the onion into the slow cooker.

3. Whisk in the remaining ingredients from the reserved bowl, until they are both well combined. Pour this into the slow cooker, stirring thoroughly until the mixture is well covered.
4. Cover in the slow cooker and cook on either high or a low heat until the beans become tender and the liquid has thickened slightly. EGANThis can take about 6 hours. Taste and then season with salt and pepper if desired.

Serves: **8-10**
Calories (Total): 996kcal 45%. Carbohydrates: 212g 77%. Protein: 40g 37%. Fat: 3.2g 4%. Saturated Fat: 0.5g 2%. Cholesterol: 0g 0%. Sodium: 3662mg 244%. Fiber: 49g 196%. Sugar: 88g 160%. Vitamin A: 1120mg 22%. Vitamin C: 28mg 38%. Calcium: 355mg 35%. Iron: 11.3mg 63%. Potassium: 2223mg 47%.

Broccoli Toasted With Garlic And Hazelnuts

This broccoli side dish has a distinctive nutty taste and is a good accompaniment to a variety of Asian dishes.

Ingredients

2 pounds broccoli florets
1 cup large raw hazelnuts
1 head garlic, peeled (12 cloves)

2 lemons, juiced
2 tablespoons olive oil
½ teaspoon kosher salt
½ teaspoon pepper

Method:
1. A 4 quart crockpot should be used for best results. First, wash and trim the broccoli, then add it to the crockpot. Peel the garlic and add in the salt and pepper. Add in the hazelnuts, squeezing in the lemon juice over the top. Toss together using wooden spoons.
2. Cover the crockpot and cook on a high heat for 2 hours, or for 4 hours on a low heat. The cooking is finished once the broccoli has reached the desired level of tenderness.

Serves: 2
Calories (Total): 775kcal 35%. Carbohydrates: 50g 18%. Protein: 26g 23%. Fat: 47g 64%. Saturated Fat: 5.8g 24%. Cholesterol: 0mg 0%. Sodium: 647mg 43%. Fiber: 25g 101%. Sugar: 24g 43%. Vitamin A: 211IU 4%. Vitamin C: 565mg 753%. Calcium: 68mg 7%. Iron: 1.1mg 6%. Potassium: 11mg 2%.

Part 2

1. Chili

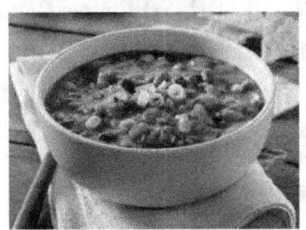

Preparation Time: 6 hours

Number of Servings: 8

Ingredients:

- 1 cup Pinto Beans
- 1 cup Black Beans
- 1 cup Kidney Beans
- 1 cup Garbanzo Beans
- 1 cup Corn
- 1/2 teaspoon Cayenne Pepper
- 1 teaspoon Cumin
- 1 tablespoon Cinnamon
- 2 tablespoon Cocoa
- 3 cloves Garlic, minced
- 3 Large Cans of Tomatoes
- 1 Dark Beer
- 1 Red Bell Pepper
- 1 White Onion
- 1 Small Can Tomato Paste

Instructions:

1) Chop up all of the veggies including the canned tomatoes and throw them all in a medium saucepan. Pour the beer, all of the spices and the tomato paste into the saucepan and bring to a boil.

2) Simmer the mixture on low for 10 minutes, then transfer it to your slow cooker.

3) Add the remaining ingredients and cook on low for 5-6 hours.

Nutritional Values (Per Serving):
- Calories 400
- Calories from Fat 26
- Total Fat 2.9g 5%
- Saturated Fat 0.5g 3%
- Trans Fat 0.0g
- Cholesterol 0mg 0%
- Sodium 66mg 3%
- Total Carbohydrates 71.7g 24%
- Dietary Fiber 18.0g 72%
- Sugars 6.1g
- Protein 22.4g
- Vitamin A 16%
- Vitamin C 49%
- Calcium 13%
- Iron 39%

2. Black Bean And Quinoa Soup

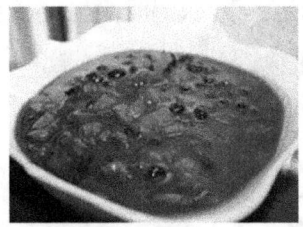

Preparation Time: 8 hours

Number of Servings: 6

Ingredients:

- 2 Dried Chipotle Peppers
- 1 lb Dried Black Beans, rinsed
- 3/4 cup Uncooked Quinoa, rinsed
- 4 Large Tomatoes
- 1 Red Onion
- 3 cloves Garlic, minced
- 1 Green Bell Pepper
- 1 Red Bell Pepper
- 1/2 tablespoon Cinnamon
- 2 teaspoons Chile Powder
- 1 teaspoon Ground Coriander
- 7 cups Water

Instructions:

1) Chop the tomatoes, onion, and peppers and add them to your slow cooker.
2) Add the remaining ingredients and stir.
3) Cook on low for 8-10 hours.

Nutritional Values (Per Serving):
- Calories 384
- Calories from Fat 24
- Total Fat 2.7g 4%
- Trans Fat 0.0g
- Cholesterol 0mg 0%
- Sodium 85mg 4%
- Total Carbohydrates 71.5g 24%
- Dietary Fiber 16.2g 65%
- Sugars 8.0g
- Protein 21.2g
- Vitamin A 49%
- Vitamin C 178%
- Calcium 13%
- Iron 40%

3. Leek And Potato Soup

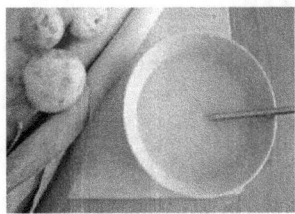

Preparation Time: 7 hours
Number of Servings: 6

Ingredients:
- 2 Leeks
- 4 Large Potatoes
- 3 Carrots, peeled
- 2 Celery Stalks
- 3 cloves Garlic, minced
- 5 cups Vegetable Broth
- 1/2 teaspoon Black Pepper

Instructions:
1) Trim and slice the leeks into small, equally sized pieces. Chop the potatoes, carrots and celery into equally sized pieces as well.
2) Add all of the ingredients to your slow cooker and cover and cook for 6 hours on low.
3) After 6 hours have passed, remove half of the soup and puree it in your food processor or blender. Return the pureed soup to your slow cooker and stir to combine.

Nutritional Values (Per Serving):

- Calories 236
- Calories from Fat 14
- Total Fat 1.6g 2%
- Trans Fat 0.0g
- Cholesterol 0mg 0%
- Sodium 683mg 28%
- Total Carbohydrates 47.3g 16%
- Dietary Fiber 7.5g 30%
- Sugars 6.1g
- Protein 9.1g
- Vitamin A 16%
- Vitamin C 93%
- Calcium 5%
- Iron 16%

4. Minestrone Soup

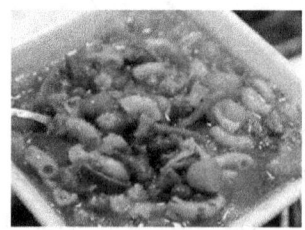

Preparation Time: 8 hours
Number of Servings: 6

Ingredients:
- 1/2 White Onion
- 1 cup Carrots
- 1 Celery Stalk
- 3 cloves Garlic, minced
- 2 Tomatoes
- 1 cup Navy Beans, rinsed
- 3 cups Vegetable Broth
- 1/4 cup Fresh Italian Basil
- 1 Sprig Fresh Rosemary
- 2 Bay Leaves
- 1 Zucchini
- 2 cups Spinach
- 2 cups Cooked Elbow Pasta

Instructions:

1) In your blender, puree the navy beans and one cup of vegetable broth together. Add the puree to your slow cooker.

2) Next, chop all of the vegetables and add them all except the zucchini and spinach to your slow cooker. Also add the garlic, vegetable broth, italian basil, rosemary, and bay leaves.

3) Cover and cook on low for 6 hours, then add the zucchini and spinach. Cook for another 30 minutes, then add the cooked pasta and stir. Allow the soup to cook for another 5-10 minutes, then remove the rosemary and bay leaves. Re-season with salt and pepper if needed then serve.

Nutritional Values (Per Serving):
- Calories 288

- Calories from Fat 22
- Total Fat 2.4g 4%
- Trans Fat 0.0g
- Cholesterol 31mg 10%
- Sodium 423mg 18%
- Total Carbohydrates 51.1g 17%
- Dietary Fiber 10.3g 41%
- Sugars 4.7g
- Protein 16.4g
- Vitamin A 31%
- Vitamin C 31%
- Calcium 8%
- Iron 28%

5. Lentil And Barley Soup

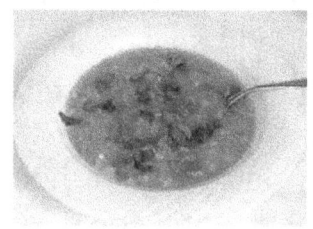

Preparation Time: 13 hours
Number of Servings: 6

Ingredients:

- 1 cup Lentils
- 1/3 cup Barley
- 1 cup Carrot, chopped
- 1 cup Celery, chopped
- 1 cup White Onion, chopped
- 2 cups Tomatoes, chopped
- 1 cup Frozen Spinach
- 3 cloves Garlic, minced
- 1/2 teaspoon Dried Basil
- 1/2 teaspoon Dried Oregano
- 1/2 teaspoon Dried Thyme
- 4 cups Vegetable Broth
- 2 cups Water

Instructions:

1) Sift through the lentils to look for any debris, then rinse them and add them to your slow cooker. Add the remaining ingredients and stir to combine.
2) Cover and cook on low for 12 hours.
Nutritional Values (Per Serving):
- Calories 206
- Calories from Fat 15
- Total Fat 1.7g 3%
- Trans Fat 0.0g
- Cholesterol 0mg 0%
- Sodium 550mg 23%
- Total Carbohydrates 34.2g 11%

- Dietary Fiber 13.6g 54%
- Sugars 4.6g
- Protein 13.9g
- Vitamin A 23%
- Vitamin C 26%
- Calcium 5%
- Iron 26%

6. Split Pea Soup

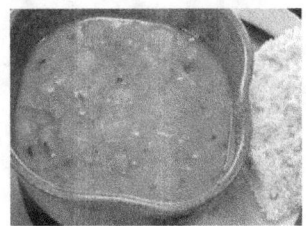

Preparation Time: 7 hours
Number of Servings: 6

Ingredients:

- 3 cups Water
- 3 cups Vegetable Broth
- 2 cups Split Peas
- 1 Stalk Celery, chopped
- 1 Large Carrot, peeled and chopped
- 1 White Onion, chopped
- 1/2 teaspoon Thyme
- 1/2 teaspoon Red Pepper Flakes
- 1 teaspoon Black Pepper

Instructions:

1) After chopping up all of the veggies, add them to your slow cooker then pour the remaining ingredients on top. Stir to combine.

2) Cover and cook on low for 6-7 hours.

Nutritional Values (Per Serving):

- Calories 258
- Calories from Fat 14
- Total Fat 1.5g 2%
- Trans Fat 0.0g
- Cholesterol 0mg 0%
- Sodium 406mg 17%
- Total Carbohydrates 43.4g 14%
- Dietary Fiber 17.7g 71%
- Sugars 7.0g
- Protein 18.9g
- Vitamin A 6%
- Vitamin C 9%
- Calcium 5%
- Iron 20%

7. Black Bean Soup

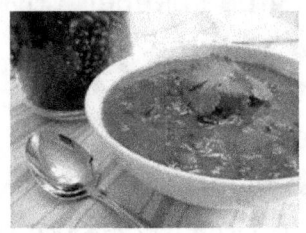

Preparation Time: 8 hours
Number of Servings: 6

Ingredients:

- 1 tablespoon Olive Oil
- 1 Yellow Onion, chopped
- 1 Large Carrot, peeled and chopped
- 1 Green Pepper, chopped
- 3 cloves Garlic, minced
- 2 cans Black Beans, drained and rinsed
- 1 can Diced Tomatoes
- 4 cups Vegetable Broth
- 1 teaspoon Ground Cumin
- 1 teaspoon Dried Thyme
- 1/2 teaspoon Dried Basil
- 1/2 teaspoon Cayenne Pepper

Instructions:

1) In a large skillet add the olive oil and the yellow onion, carrot, and green pepper. Cover and cook for 3-5 minutes, then add the minced garlic. Cook for another 2-3 minutes.

2) Transfer the veggies to your slow cooker then add the remaining ingredients.

3) Cover and cook on low for 7-8 hours.

Nutritional Values (Per Serving):

- Calories 517
- Calories from Fat 48
- Total Fat 5.4g 8%
- Saturated Fat 1.1g 5%
- Trans Fat 0.0g
- Cholesterol 0mg 0%
- Sodium 528mg 22%
- Total Carbohydrates 87.8g 29%
- Dietary Fiber 21.5g 86%
- Sugars 6.4g
- Protein 32.2g
- Vitamin A 13%
- Vitamin C 45%
- Calcium 18%
- Iron 47%

8. Vegan Ratatouille

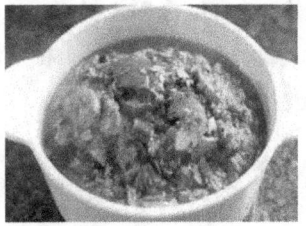

Preparation Time: 4 hours

Number of Servings: 6

Ingredients:

- 1 Eggplant, peeled and cut into cubes
- 2 Yellow Onions, chopped
- 3 Tomatoes, chopped
- 1 Green Bell Pepper, chopped
- 2 Zucchini, diced
- 3 tablespoons Olive Oil
- 3 cloves Garlic, minced
- 1 small Can Tomato Paste
- Salt and Pepper

Instructions:

1) Lay the eggplant out on a wire wrack and sprinkle with salt. Let the eggplant cubes sit for 1/2 an hour to draw the extra water out of them.

2) After the water has drained from the eggplant, rinse the salt off of the cubes and add them to your slow cooker.

3) Add the onions, bell pepper, zucchini, tomatoes, and garlic. Season with salt and pepper and mix well. Pour the olive oil over the veggies and stir.

4) Cover and cook for 3 hours on low.

5) Stir the tomato paste into the fully cooked veggies and serve.

Nutritional Values (Per Serving):

- Calories 122
- Calories from Fat 67
- Total Fat 7.5g 12%
- Saturated Fat 1.1g 5%
- Cholesterol 0mg 0%
- Sodium 12mg 1%
- Total Carbohydrates 13.6g 5%
- Dietary Fiber 5.3g 21%
- Sugars 6.9g
- Protein 2.5g
- Vitamin A 25%
- Vitamin C 88%
- Calcium 1%
- Iron 13%

9. Sweet And Spicy Curry

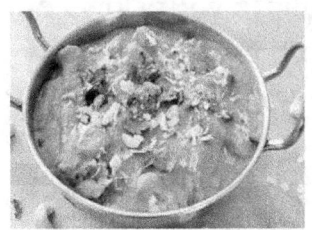

Preparation Time: 7 hours
Number of Servings: 6

Ingredients:

- 2 tablespoon Olive Oil
- 1 White Onion, chopped
- 4 Stalks Celery, chopped
- 1/3 Head Cabbage, shredded
- 1 Sweet Potato, diced
- 1 can Chickpeas, rinsed
- 3 cups Vegetable Broth
- 1 can Coconut Milk
- 1 teaspoon Garlic Powder
- 1 teaspoon Cayenne Pepper
- 1 teaspoon Cinnamon
- 1 teaspoon Ground Ginger
- 1 teaspoon Curry Powder
- Salt and Pepper

Instructions:

1) Pour the olive oil into your slow cooker and coat the bottom and sides of the slow cooker with the oil.
2) Add the chopped white onion and all of the spices and stir.
3) Next, add the remaining ingredients, except the coconut milk, and mix well.
4) Cover and cook on low for 6 hours.
5) 20 minutes before the curry is finished add the coconut milk and stir. Re-season the curry with salt and pepper then allow it to cook for the remaining time period.
6) Serve plain or with rice.

Nutritional Values (Per Serving):

- Calories 401
- Calories from Fat 239
- Total Fat 26.5g 41%
- Saturated Fat 18.0g 90%
- Trans Fat 0.0g
- Cholesterol 0mg 0%
- Sodium 425mg 18%
- Total Carbohydrates 33.4g 11%
- Dietary Fiber 9.7g 39%
- Sugars 10.1g
- Protein 11.8g
- Vitamin A 75%

- Vitamin C 41%
- Calcium 8%
- Iron 22%

10. Bean And Spinach Enchiladas

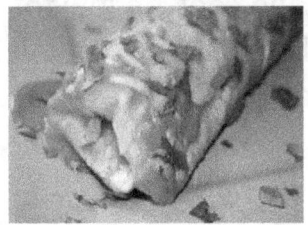

Preparation Time: 4 hours

Number of Servings: 4

Ingredients:
- 1 can Black Beans, drained and rinsed
- 2 cups Frozen Spinach, thawed and drained
- 1 cup Frozen Corn
- 1/2 teaspoon Ground Cumin
- 2 cups Salsa
- 6 cups Romaine Lettuce, chopped
- 4 Radishes, chopped
- 1/2 cup Cherry Tomatoes, sliced
- 1/2 Cucumber, diced
- 8 Vegan Tortillas

Instructions:

1) Pour 1 cup of salsa into your slow cooker and coat the bottom of the slow cooker with it.
2) Next, in a small bowl add the beans, corn, spinach, and cumin powder and mix. Scoop this mixture into the tortillas and then carefully roll them up.
3) Lay the tortillas on top of the slow cooker with their seams down. Pour the remaining cup of salsa over the tortillas then cover and cook on low for 3 hours.
4) Top the cooked enchiladas with lettuce, radishes, cherry tomatoes, and cucumbers to serve.

Nutritional Values (Per Serving):

- Calories 527
- Calories from Fat 32
- Total Fat 3.6g 5%
- Saturated Fat 0.7g 4%
- Trans Fat 0.0g
- Cholesterol 0mg 0%
- Sodium 831mg 35%
- Total Carbohydrates 102.9g 34%
- Dietary Fiber 22.6g 90%
- Sugars 9.9g
- Protein 28.3g
- Vitamin A 47%
- Vitamin C 26%
- Calcium 23%
- Iron 50%

11. Mushroom Stroganoff

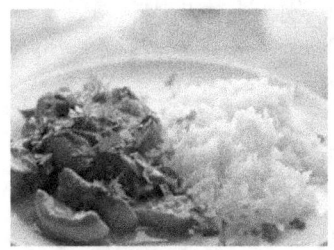

Preparation Time: 8 hours
Number of Servings: 4

Ingredients:

- 4 cups Mushrooms, sliced
- 1 White Onion, diced
- 1 tablespoon Vegan Butter Spread
- 2 tablespoon Tomato Ketchup
- 2 1/2 cups Vegetable Broth
- 3 teaspoon Smoked Paprika
- 3 cloves Garlic, minced
- 4 tablespoons Plain Vegan Yogurt

Instructions:

1) In a large skillet, melt the vegan butter spread and cook the onions and mushrooms for 10 minutes over low heat.

2) Transfer this mixture to your slow cooker and add the remaining ingredients. Stir well to combine.
3) Cook on low for 7-8 hours.
4) Serve with pasta, rice or plain.

Nutritional Values (Per Serving):

- Calories 66
- Calories from Fat 12
- Total Fat 1.3g 2%
- Cholesterol 0mg 0%
- Sodium 565mg 24%
- Total Carbohydrates 8.9g 3%
- Dietary Fiber 1.9g 8%
- Sugars 4.7g
- Protein 5.9g
- Vitamin A 18%
- Vitamin C 15%
- Calcium 1%
- Iron 15%

12. Lentil Taco Filling

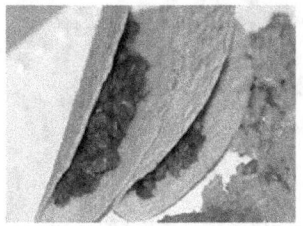

Preparation Time: 8 hours
Number of Servings: 6

Ingredients:

- 1/2 cup Brown Lentils
- 1/4 cup Quinoa, rinsed
- 2 cups Water
- 3 cloves Garlic, minced
- 1/2 teaspoon Chili Powder
- 1/2 teaspoon Paprika
- 1 tablespoon Taco Seasoning

Instructions:

1) Add all of the ingredients to your slow cooker and cover and cook on low for 7-8 hours.
2) Serve with taco shells or on lettuce for a taco salad.

Nutritional Values (Per Serving):

- Calories 113
- Calories from Fat 35
- Total Fat 3.9g 6%
- Saturated Fat 1.9g 10%
- Trans Fat 0.0g
- Cholesterol 9mg 3%
- Sodium 141mg 6%
- Total Carbohydrates 15.8g 5%
- Dietary Fiber 3.6g 15%
- Protein 7.2g
- Vitamin A 6%
- Vitamin C 2%
- Calcium 5%
- Iron 9%

13. Fajitas Filling

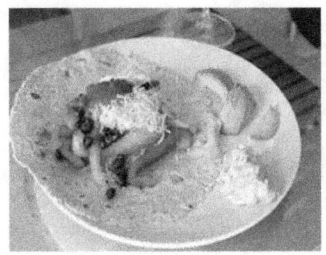

Preparation Time: 5 hours
Number of Servings: 8

Ingredients:

- 3 Tomatoes, diced
- 1 Green Bell Pepper, sliced
- 1 Red Bell Pepper, sliced
- 1 White Onion, sliced
- 2 teaspoons Cumin
- 2 teaspoons Chili Powder
- 2 cloves Garlic, minced
- 1 tablespoon Olive Oil

Instructions:

1) Pour the olive oil in your slow cooker and coat the bottom and sides of the pot with the oil.

2) Add all of the ingredients and stir to combine.
3) Cook on low for 4-5 hours. Serve with tortillas or eat plain.

Nutritional Values (Per Serving):

- Calories 44
- Calories from Fat 19
- Total Fat 2.1g 3%
- Cholesterol 0mg 0%
- Sodium 11mg 0%
- Total Carbohydrates 5.7g 2%
- Dietary Fiber 1.8g 7%
- Sugars 3.1g
- Protein 1.0g
- Vitamin A 30%
- Vitamin C 78%
- Calcium 1%
- Iron 7%

14. Non-Fried Refried Beans

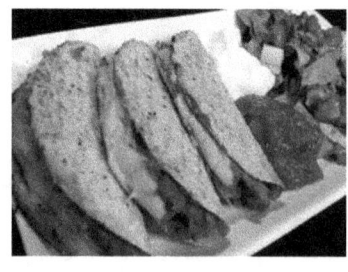

Preparation Time: 11 hours
Number of Servings: 15

Ingredients:

- 1 White Onion, chopped
- 3 cups Dried Pinto Beans, rinsed
- 1 Jalapeño Pepper, chopped
- 3 cloves Garlic, minced
- 2 teaspoons Salt
- 2 teaspoons Black Pepper
- 1/2 teaspoon Ground Cumin
- 4 cups Water
- 5 cups Vegetable Broth

Instructions:

1) Place all of the dried ingredients into the slow cooker and then pour the water and vegetable broth over these ingredients. Stir well to combine.
2) Cook on low for 10 hours then drain the beans and reserve the liquid. Mash the beans with a fork or a potato masher and add some of the reserved water to keep the consistency smooth. Serve on tortilla shells.

Nutritional Values (Per Serving):

- Calories 152

- Calories from Fat 9
- Total Fat 1.0g 1%
- Cholesterol 0mg 0%
- Sodium 571mg 24%
- Total Carbohydrates 25.5g 9%
- Dietary Fiber 6.2g 25%
- Sugars 1.4g
- Protein 10.0g
- Vitamin A 0%
- Vitamin C 6%
- Calcium 5%
- Iron 13%

15. Slow Cooker Spicy Chickpeas

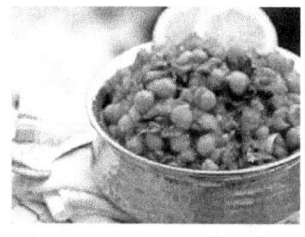

Preparation Time: 8 hours

Number of Servings: 6

Ingredients:

- 1 tablespoon Olive Oil
- 2 White Onions, diced
- 5 cloves Garlic, minced
- 2 teaspoons Ground Coriander
- 1 teaspoon Cumin
- 1 teaspoon Salt
- 1 teaspoon Black Pepper
- 1/4 teaspoon Cayenne Pepper
- 1 Tomato, diced
- 2 Cans Chickpeas, rinsed and drained

Instructions:

1) In a skillet, add the olive oil and onion. Cook the onion until it is translucent then add the minced garlic. Cook for 2-3 minutes.
2) Transfer the onion and garlic mixture to your slow cooker and add the remaining ingredients, stirring well to combine.
3) Cook on low for 7 hours.
4) Serve with tortillas, bread or pita.

Nutritional Values (Per Serving):

- Calories 527
- Calories from Fat 94
- Total Fat 10.5g 16%
- Saturated Fat 1.2g 6%
- Cholesterol 0mg 0%

- Sodium 421mg 18%
- Total Carbohydrates 85.5g 29%
- Dietary Fiber 24.2g 97%
- Sugars 15.9g
- Protein 26.3g
- Vitamin A 3%
- Vitamin C 19%
- Calcium 15%
- Iron 48%

16. Mediterranean Vegetables With Beans

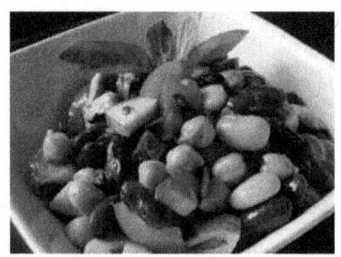

Preparation Time: 8 hours
Number of Servings: 6

Ingredients:

- 1 can Navy Beans, drained and rinsed
- 1 can Red Beans, drained and rinsed
- 2 cloves Garlic, minced

- 1 White Onion, chopped
- 1 Large Carrot, peeled and chopped
- 2 Celery Stalks, diced
- 2 cups Green Beans
- Salt and Pepper

Instructions:

1) Add all of the ingredients to your slow cooker and season with salt and pepper.
2) Cook on low for 8 hours.

Nutritional Values (Per Serving):

- Calories 467
- Calories from Fat 16
- Total Fat 1.8g 3%
- Trans Fat 0.0g
- Cholesterol 0mg 0%
- Sodium 26mg 1%
- Total Carbohydrates 85.7g 29%
- Dietary Fiber 28.3g 113%
- Sugars 6.0g
- Protein 30.3g
- Vitamin A 8%
- Vitamin C 25%
- Calcium 17%
- Iron 47%

17. Sweet Potato Risotto

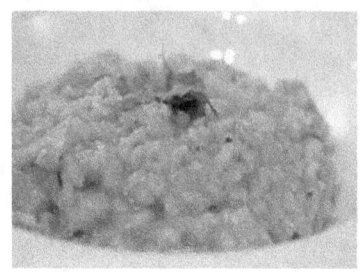

Preparation Time: 8 hours
Number of Servings: 6

Ingredients:

- 1/2 tablespoon Extra Virgin Olive Oil
- 2 cloves Garlic, minced
- 1/2 teaspoon Dried Rosemary
- 1 1/2 cups Pearl Barley
- 2 cups Vegetable Broth
- 1 cup Water
- 2 Large Sweet Potatoes, peeled and diced

Instructions:

1) In a large skillet, heat the extra virgin olive oil and then add the onions and cook until they are translucent.

2) Add the garlic and rosemary and cook for another minute.

3) Next, add the barley and stir to coat the barley in onions, garlic and rosemary. Add the vegetable broth and water and bring the mixture to a boil.

4) Place your diced sweet potatoes in the bottom of your slow cooker then pour the boiling barley mixture over the potatoes.

5) Cover and cook for 8 hours on low.

Nutritional Values (Per Serving):

- Calories 260
- Calories from Fat 21
- Total Fat 2.3g 4%
- Cholesterol 0mg 0%
- Sodium 265mg 11%
- Total Carbohydrates 53.5g 18%
- Dietary Fiber 9.9g 40%
- Sugars 0.9g
- Protein 7.4g
- Vitamin A 2%
- Vitamin C 15%
- Calcium 3%
- Iron 10%

18. Red Beans And Barley

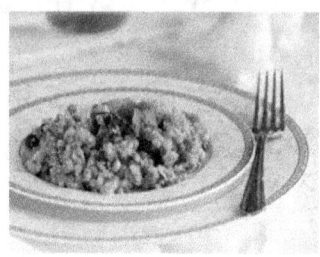

Preparation Time: 8 hours
Number of Servings: 6

Ingredients:

- 1 cup Uncooked Barley
- 1 Red Onion, diced
- 1 Stalk Celery, diced
- 2 cloves Garlic, minced
- 1/2 teaspoon Red Pepper Flakes
- 1 can Kidney Beans, rinsed and drained
- 2 Tomatoes, diced
- 3 cups Vegetable Broth
- 1 teaspoon Black Pepper

Instructions:

1) Place all of the ingredients in your slow cooker and cover and cook for 7-8 hours on low.

Nutritional Values (Per Serving):

- Calories 353
- Calories from Fat 20
- Total Fat 2.2g 3%
- Trans Fat 0.0g
- Cholesterol 0mg 0%
- Sodium 397mg 17%
- Total Carbohydrates 64.6g 22%
- Dietary Fiber 15.7g 63%
- Sugars 3.8g
- Protein 20.7g
- Vitamin A 8%
- Vitamin C 19%
- Calcium 7%
- Iron 35%

19. Slow Cooker Greens

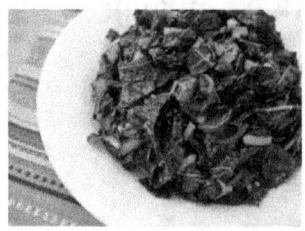

Preparation Time: 3 hours 30 minutes
Number of Servings: 6

Ingredients:

- 2 tablespoons Olive Oil
- 1/2 cup White Onion
- 4 cloves Garlic, minced
- 2 cups Kale
- 2 cups Collard Greens
- 1/2 cup Parsley
- 1 can Black Beans
- 2 teaspoons Herbs de Provence
- 1/2 teaspoon Black Pepper
- 1 cup Vegetable Broth

Instructions:

1) Add the garlic, onion and olive oil to your slow cooker and turn the heat on high. Stir the ingredients to coat the bottom of the slow cooker. Cover the slow cooker and continue cooking the mixture on high for 10 minutes.

2) Chop up the greens and toss them all into your slow cooker. Stir well to combine then add the remaining ingredients. Stir again, then cover and cook on high for 1 hour. Reduce the heat to low and continue cooking for 2 hours.

Nutritional Values (Per Serving):

- Calories 291
- Calories from Fat 56
- Total Fat 6.2g 10%
- Saturated Fat 1.0g 5%
- Trans Fat 0.0g
- Cholesterol 0mg 0%
- Sodium 145mg 6%
- Total Carbohydrates 45.2g 15%
- Dietary Fiber 11.6g 46%
- Sugars 2.5g
- Protein 16.4g
- Vitamin A 63%
- Vitamin C 67%
- Calcium 14%
- Iron 23%

20. Winter Stew

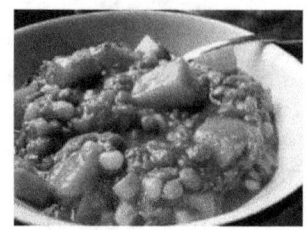

Preparation Time: 7 hours
Number of Servings: 6

Ingredients:

- 4 cups Mushroom Broth
- 4 cups Water
- 5 Red Potatoes, diced
- 2 Yellow Onions, diced
- 5 cloves Garlic, minced
- 2 Large Carrots, peeled and chopped
- 2 Tomatoes, diced
- 1 tablespoon Dried Oregano
- 1/2 tablespoon Dried Parsley
- 1/4 teaspoon Smoked Paprika
- 1 teaspoon Salt
- 1 teaspoon Black Pepper
- 1 Dark Beer
- 1 cup Portobello Mushrooms, diced
- 1 cup Corn

Instructions:

1) After chopping and dicing all of the vegetables add all of the ingredients except the corn and portobello mushrooms to your slow cooker.
2) Cover and cook for 5-6 hours.
3) Half an hour before serving add the portobello mushrooms and corn and continue cooking.

Nutritional Values (Per Serving):

- Calories 214
- Calories from Fat 6
- Total Fat 0.7g 1%
- Trans Fat 0.0g
- Cholesterol 0mg 0%
- Sodium 778mg 32%
- Total Carbohydrates 44.9g 15%
- Dietary Fiber 6.1g 24%
- Sugars 6.4g
- Protein 5.5g
- Vitamin A 14%
- Vitamin C 53%
- Calcium 4%
- Iron 20%

21. Stuffed Zucchini

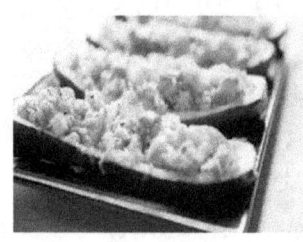

Preparation Time: 5 hours 30 minutes
Number of Servings: 2

Ingredients:

- 1 Medium Zucchini
- 1 cup Marinara Sauce
- 1 White Onion, chopped
- 2 cloves Garlic, minced
- 1/4 cup Uncooked Brown Rice
- 1 tablespoon Dried Parsley
- 1 tablespoon Dried Basil
- 1 teaspoon Black Pepper

Instructions:

1) In a small mixing bowl combine the onions, garlic, brown rice, spices and 2 tablespoons of the marinara sauce. Mix well.

2) Cut the zucchini in half lengthwise and remove any visible seeds. Scoop out some of the flesh then pour the onion and rice mixture into each zucchini half.

3) Place the zucchini in your slow cooker and cover with the remaining marinara sauce.

4) Cover and cook on low for 4-6 hours, or until the rice has cooked all of the way through.

Nutritional Values (Per Serving):

- Calories 238
- Calories from Fat 38
- Total Fat 4.2g 6%
- Saturated Fat 1.0g 5%
- Trans Fat 0.0g
- Cholesterol 3mg 1%
- Sodium 524mg 22%
- Total Carbohydrates 44.7g 15%
- Dietary Fiber 6.4g 26%
- Sugars 15.1g
- Protein 5.8g
- Vitamin A 16%
- Vitamin C 47%
- Calcium 6%
- Iron 10%

22. Almond Barley Casserole

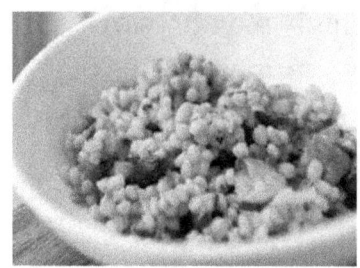

Preparation Time: 8 hours
Number of Servings: 5

Ingredients:

- 1 cup Uncooked Barley
- 1 1/2 cups V8 Vegetable Juice
- 1/2 teaspoon Black Pepper
- 2 Celery Stalks, chopped
- 1 Red Bell Pepper, chopped
- 1 White Onion, chopped
- 2 cups Vegetable Broth
- 1/4 cup Almonds, toasted

Instructions:

1) To toast the almonds add them to a nonstick skillet and cook them over medium heat for 5 minutes, or until browned.

2) Next, mix all of the ingredients except the almonds in your slow cooker and cover and cook for 6-8 hours on low.

3) Stir in the toasted almonds before serving.

Nutritional Values (Per Serving):

- Calories 191
- Calories from Fat 35
- Total Fat 3.8g 6%
- Saturated Fat 0.5g 3%
- Trans Fat 0.0g
- Cholesterol 0mg 0%
- Sodium 316mg 13%
- Total Carbohydrates 32.2g 11%
- Dietary Fiber 8.1g 32%
- Sugars 2.8g
- Protein 8.0g
- Vitamin A 16%
- Vitamin C 56%
- Calcium 3%
- Iron 10%

23. Pineapple Barbecue Tofu

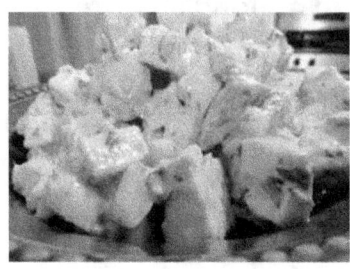

Preparation Time: 8 hours
Number of Servings: 6

Ingredients:

- 2 Packages Extra Firm Tofu, frozen and defrosted
- 1 White Onion, chopped
- 6 cloves Garlic, minced
- 1 1/2 cup Crushed Pineapple
- 1/3 cup Water
- 3 tablespoons Ginger, minced
- 5 tablespoons Tomato Paste
- 2 tablespoons Soy Sauce
- 1 tablespoon Lemon Juice
- 1 teaspoon Black Pepper

Instructions:

1) Cut the defrosted tofu into 1/2 inch cubes and then add them to your slow cooker.
2) Next, in a medium skillet sauté the onion for 3-5 minutes, then add the minced garlic and cook for 1 more minute. Transfer this mixture to your blender and add the remaining ingredients to your blender. Blend until smooth.
3) Pour the blended mixture over your tofu and stir.
4) Cover and cook on low for 7-8 hours.

Nutritional Values (Per Serving):

- Calories 146
- Calories from Fat 50
- Total Fat 5.6g 9%
- Saturated Fat 1.2g 6%
- Trans Fat 0.0g
- Cholesterol 0mg 0%
- Sodium 332mg 14%
- Total Carbohydrates 15.4g 5%
- Dietary Fiber 3.2g 13%
- Sugars 7.5g
- Protein 12.1g
- Vitamin A 5%
- Vitamin C 46%
- Calcium 27%
- Iron 17%

24. Wild Rice

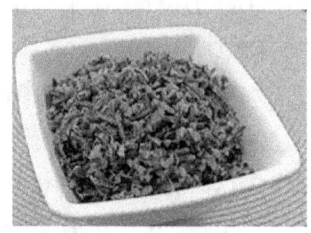

Preparation Time: 4 hours
Number of Servings: 6
Ingredients:

- 2 1/2 cups Vegetable Broth
- 1 cup Wild Rice
- 2 cloves Garlic, minced
- 1 Yellow Onion, diced
- 1 Stalk Celery, diced
- 1/2 teaspoon Dried Parsley
- 1/2 teaspoon Salt
- 1 teaspoon Black Pepper

Instructions:

1) Add all of the ingredients to your slow cooker and stir to combine.
2) Cover and cook on low for 4 hours.

Nutritional Values (Per Serving):

- Calories 122
- Calories from Fat 8
- Total Fat 0.9g 1%
- Trans Fat 0.0g
- Cholesterol 0mg 0%
- Sodium 516mg 22%
- Total Carbohydrates 22.7g 8%
- Dietary Fiber 2.2g 9%
- Sugars 1.8g
- Protein 6.2g
- Vitamin A 1%
- Vitamin C 5%
- Calcium 1%
- Iron 5%

25. Chai Pear Applesauce

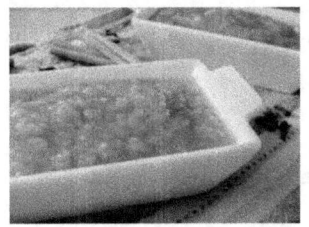

Preparation Time: 6 hours 30 minutes
Number of Servings: 6

Ingredients:

- 4 Red Apples, peeled, cored and chopped
- 4 Pears, peeled, cored and chopped
- 1 teaspoon Lemon Juice
- 2 tablespoons Brown Sugar
- 1/2 tablespoon Cinnamon
- 1/2 teaspoon Ground Ginger
- 1/2 teaspoon Ground Cloves
- 1/2 teaspoon Nutmeg

Instructions:

1) Add all of the ingredients to your slow cooker and stir to combine.

2) Cover and cook on low for 6 hours, stirring every hour to break down the fruit. Puree the applesauce if you do not want chunks of fruit in the final product.

Nutritional Values (Per Serving):

- Calories 159
- Calories from Fat 3
- Total Fat 0.3g 0%
- Trans Fat 0.0g
- Cholesterol 0mg 0%
- Sodium 4mg 0%
- Total Carbohydrates 42.0g 14%

- Dietary Fiber 7.6g 31%
- Sugars 29.3g
- Protein 0.6g
- Vitamin A 2%
- Vitamin C 20%
- Calcium 3%
- Iron 3%

26. Maple Brown Sugar Oatmeal

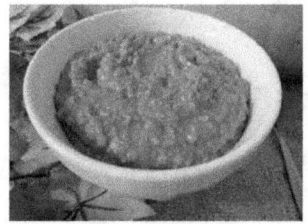

Preparation Time: 8 hours

Number of Servings: 6

Ingredients:

- 5 cups Water
- 1 cup Almond, Rice or Soy Milk
- 2 cups Steel Cut Oats
- 1/4 cup Maple Syrup
- 1/4 cup Brown Sugar
- 2 teaspoons Cinnamon

Instructions:

1) Combine all of the ingredients in your slow cooker and stir to mix well.
2) Cover and cook on low for 8 hours.

Nutritional Values (Per Serving):

- Calories 185
- Calories from Fat 23
- Total Fat 2.5g 4%
- Trans Fat 0.0g
- Cholesterol 0mg 0%
- Sodium 31mg 1%
- Total Carbohydrates 36.4g 12%
- Dietary Fiber 3.4g 14%
- Sugars 15.6g
- Protein 5.0g
- Vitamin A 0%
- Vitamin C 0%
- Calcium 5%
- Iron 9%

27. Lemon Blueberry Cake

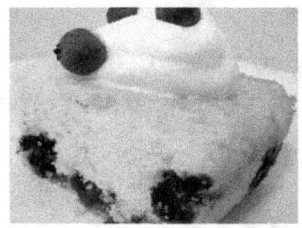

Preparation Time: 1 hour 30 minutes
Number of Servings: 4

Ingredients:

- 1/2 cup Whole Wheat Flour
- 1/2 teaspoon Agave Nectar
- 1/4 teaspoon Baking Powder
- 1/3 cup Plain Soy Milk
- 1/4 cup Fresh or Frozen Blueberries, defrosted if using frozen
- 1 teaspoon Ground Flaxseeds
- 2 teaspoons Warm Water
- 1/2 teaspoon Lemon Zest
- 1 teaspoon Applesauce
- 1/2 teaspoon Vanilla Extract
- 1/4 teaspoon Lemon Extract

Instructions:

1) Line your slow cooker with parchment paper.
2) Next, mix together the wheat flour, baking powder and agave nectar.
3) In a small bowl mix together the warm water and ground flaxseeds. Next, mix the remaining ingredients into the flaxseed mixture.
4) Combine the wet and dry ingredients then pour the mixture into your slow cooker.
5) Place a clean towel over your slow cooker then carefully set the lid on top.
6) Cook on high for 60-70 minutes.

Nutritional Values (Per Serving):
Calories 79

Calories from Fat 7

Total Fat 0.7g 1%

Trans Fat 0.0g

Cholesterol 0mg 0%

Sodium 11mg 0%

Total Carbohydrates 15.0g 5%

Dietary Fiber 1.1g 4%

Sugars 2.0g

Protein 2.5g

Vitamin A 0%

Vitamin C 3%

Calcium 2%

Iron 6%

28. Coconut Rice Pudding

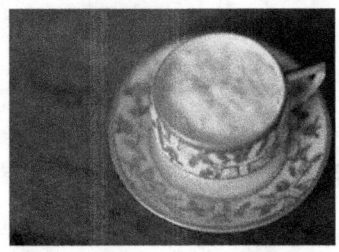

Preparation Time: 4 hours

Number of Servings: 5

Ingredients:

- 1/2 cup White Rice
- 1 can Coconut Milk
- 1 cup Vanilla Almond Milk
- 1/4 cup Water
- 1/2 teaspoon Cinnamon
- 1/4 teaspoon Almond Extract
- 1/2 teaspoon Nutmeg
- 1/4 cup Raisins
- 1/4 cup Almonds
- 1/4 cup Coconut Flakes

Instructions:

1) Add the rice, coconut milk, vanilla almond milk, almond extract, and spices to your slow cooker.
2) Cook on low for 4 hours.
3) When ready to serve, mix the raisins, almonds and coconut into the rice pudding.

Nutritional Values (Per Serving):

- Calories 372
- Calories from Fat 246
- Total Fat 27.3g 42%
- Saturated Fat 21.7g 109%
- Trans Fat 0.0g
- Cholesterol 0mg 0%
- Sodium 47mg 2%
- Total Carbohydrates 31.0g 10%
- Dietary Fiber 3.9g 16%
- Sugars 11.0g
- Protein 5.1g
- Vitamin A 2%
- Vitamin C 5%
- Calcium 10%
- Iron 19%

29. Scalloped Peaches

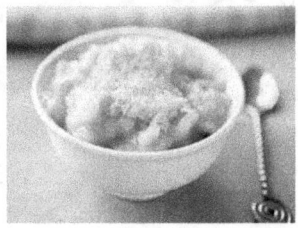

Preparation Time: 2 hours
Number of Servings: 8

Ingredients:

- 8 Peaches, sliced
- 1 cup Sugar
- 1 teaspoon Cinnamon
- 1/4 cup Vegan Butter Spread

Instructions:

1) Combine all of the ingredients in your slow cooker then cover and cook on low for 2 hours.

Nutritional Values (Per Serving):

- Calories 133
- Calories from Fat 2

- Total Fat 0.2g 0%
- Trans Fat 0.0g
- Cholesterol 0mg 0%
- Sodium 0mg 0%
- Total Carbohydrates 34.6g 12%
- Dietary Fiber 1.6g 6%
- Sugars 33.2g
- Protein 0.9g
- Vitamin A 6%
- Vitamin C 11%
- Calcium 1%
- Iron 2%

30. Cinnamon Applesauce

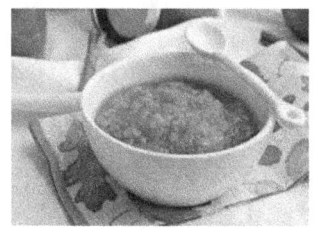

Preparation Time: 7 hours
Number of Servings: 6

Ingredients:

- 5 Red Delicious Apples, cored, peeled and chopped
- 5 Golden Delicious Apples, cored, peeled and chopped
- 1 tablespoon Cinnamon
- 1 tablespoon Agave Nectar
- 1 teaspoon Lemon Juice

Instructions:

1) Combine all of the ingredients in your slow cooker and stir.
2) Cover and cook on low for 6-7 hours, stirring every couple of hours to break down the apples.
3) When finished, re-season with cinnamon or agave nectar to balance out the flavors.

Nutritional Values (Per Serving):

- Calories 161
- Calories from Fat 0
- Total Fat 0.0g 0%
- Trans Fat 0.0g
- Cholesterol 0mg 0%
- Sodium 3mg 0%
- Total Carbohydrates 42.8g 14%
- Dietary Fiber 7.9g 32%
- Sugars 31.6g
- Protein 0.1g
- Vitamin A 3%
- Vitamin C 24%

- Calcium 3%
- Iron 3%

Southern Style Beets

Ingredients:
½ cup raw honey
¼ cup water
¼ cup white vinegar
2 cans whole beets, drained

Directions:
Combine ingredients in the slow cooker and cook on low for 6-8 hours.

Summer Zucchini

Ingredients:
4 TBSP coconut oil
1 onion, sliced
1 cucumber, seeded and sliced
2 large zucchini, sliced
1 green bell pepper, julienned
1 red bell pepper, julienned
½ cup apple cider
Salt and pepper to taste

Directions:
Combine all ingredients in the slow cooker and cook on low for 4-6 hours or until vegetables are tender.

Greek Style Eggplant

Ingredients:
1 large eggplant, cut into 1-inch cubes
2 onions, sliced
2 celery stalks, sliced
1 TBSP olive oil
2 cans dice tomatoes with liquid
3 TBSP tomato sauce
½ cup olives, pitted and halved
2 TBSP balsamic vinegar
1 TBSP honey
1 tsp oregano
Salt and pepper to taste

Directions:
Add all ingredients to the slow cooker and stir to combine. Cook on low for 4-5 hours or until eggplant is tender.

Dinner Vegetable Medley

Ingredients:
1 medium cabbage, chopped
1 small rutabaga, cut in chunks
3 stalks of celery, chopped
2 dozen baby carrots
2 medium onions, cut in chunks
1 tsp onion powder
1 can diced tomatoes

1 can organic vegetable juice

Directions:
Combine all ingredients in the slow cooker and cover. Cook on low for 4-6 hours and serve.

Italian Stewed Tomatoes

Ingredients:
7 or 8 ripe tomatoes, diced
2 TBSP coconut oil
1 medium onion, sliced
¾ cup chopped celery
½ cup bell pepper, chopped
3 TBSP raw honey
1 tsp parsley
1/8 tsp pepper
1 tsp Salt

Directions:
Combine all ingredients in the slow cooker and stir. Cover and cook on low for 8-10 hours. Serve over rice.

Slow Cooked Artichokes

Ingredients:
5 artichokes, stalks removed
1 ½ tsp Salt
8 peppercorns

2 stalks celery, sliced
1 lemon, cut into rounds
2 cups water

Directions:
Combine all ingredients in the slow cooker and cook on low for 4-6 hours.

Stuffed Peppers

Ingredients:
4 large green bell peppers
1 cup steamed cauliflower, mashed
1 cup whole kernel corn
1 cup olives, pits removed and cut in half
½ cup chives
¼ tsp sea salt
¼ tsp garlic pepper
1 can diced tomatoes with liquid
1/3 cup red wine vinegar
1 can tomato paste

Directions:
Cut tops off peppers and scoop out seeds and inner ribs. Remove the stems from the tops and cut up remaining pepper pieces. Add pepper pieces to a mixing bowl with steamed cauliflower, corn, olives, chives, ½ diced tomatoes, and seasonings. Mix together and stuff the peppers, packing lightly. Stand the peppers upright in your slow cooker. In a separate

bowl, combine remaining tomatoes with their liquid, vinegar, and tomato paste and stir. Pour mixture over and around the peppers in the slow cooker.

Cover and cook on low for 5-6 hours until peppers are tender, but still hold their shape.

Barbecue Tofu

Ingredients:
2 containers firm or extra firm tofu, pressed
1 1/2 cups ketchup
3 TBSP brown sugar
2 TBSP soy sauce
1 TBSP apple cider vinegar
1 TBSP red pepper flakes
1/2 tsp garlic powder
Salt and pepper to taste

Directions:
Combine all ingredients in a slow cooker. Cover and cook on low for 5-6 hours.

Teriyaki Tofu

Ingredients:
2 containers firm or extra firm tofu, pressed
1 1/2 cups teriyaki sauce

1 TBSP apple cider vinegar
1/2 tsp garlic powder
Salt and pepper to taste

Directions:
Combine all ingredients in a slow cooker. Cover and cook on low for 5-6 hours.

White Beans and Sun Dried Tomatoes

Ingredients:
2 cups Great Northern beans
3 cloves garlic, minced
1 onion, chopped
3 cups vegetable broth
3 cups water
1 tsp Salt
1/2 tsp Italian seasoning
3/4 cup chopped sun dried tomatoes in oil, drained
4 ounce can sliced black olives, drained
1 cup shredded cheese substitute

Directions:
Combine all ingredients in the slow cooker except tomatoes, olives, and cheese substitute. Cover and cook on low 4-6 hours or until beans are tender. Stir in tomatoes, olives, and cheese substitute and cover. Cook for an additional hour.

Slow Cooker Ravioli

Ingredients:
1 onion, chopped
3 cloves garlic, minced
4 cups marinara sauce
8 oz. can tomato sauce
1 (14-ounce) can diced tomatoes, undrained
4 (9 oz.) packages of refrigerated vegan ravioli
2 cups shredded cheese substitute

Directions:
Place onion and garlic in bottom of 4-6 quart slow cooker. Add spaghetti sauce, tomato sauce, and undrained tomatoes and stir well. Cover and cook on low for 8-9 hours until onion is tender. Turn heat to high and stir in refrigerated ravioli. Cover and cook on high for 1 hour longer; then sprinkle with cheese substitute and cook for 5-10 minutes until ravioli is tender.

Three Bean Italian Cassoulet

Ingredients:
1 cup dried lima beans
1 cup dried great Northern beans
1 cup dried garbanzo beans
4-1/2 cups water
16 oz. bag baby carrots

1 onion, chopped
3 garlic cloves, minced
2 TBSP Italian seasoning
1/2 tsp salt
1/8 tsp white pepper
1 bay leaf
14 oz. can diced tomatoes, undrained
2 TBSP tomato paste

Directions:
Soak beans overnight and drain. Combine beans, 4-1/2 cups water, carrots, onion, garlic and seasonings except Salt, tomatoes, and tomato paste in 3-1/2 to 4 quart slow cooker. Mix well to combine. Cover and cook on high for 30 minutes. Reduce heat to low and cook for 8-9 hours or until beans and vegetables are tender. Stir in tomatoes, tomato paste, and Salt, cover, and cook 1 hour longer on low. Remove bay leaf before serving.

Barley Casserole

Ingredients:
1 TBSP olive oil
1 yellow onion, chopped
3 cloves garlic, minced
1 cup uncooked pearl barley
½ cup tomato juice
½ tsp thyme
½ tsp oregano
¼ tsp salt

¼ tsp pepper
1 red bell pepper, chopped
1 cup chopped mushrooms
2-1/2 cups vegetable broth
1/3 cup toasted pine nuts

Directions:
Saute onion and garlic in olive oil until tender. Then combine all ingredients except pine nuts in a 3-quart slow cooker. Cover and cook on low for 6-8 hours until barley and vegetables are tender. Sprinkle with nuts just before serving.

Meatless Sloppy Joes

Ingredients:
1 cup lentils, soaked overnight
2 cups water
2 onions, chopped
3 carrots, chopped
4 stalks celery, chopped
3/4 cup ketchup
3 TBSP brown sugar
1 TBSP cider vinegar
1 TBSP yellow mustard
1 tsp Italian seasoning
10 sandwich rolls, split and toasted

Directions:

Combine all ingredients except for vinegar, mustard, and sandwich rolls. Place in the slow cooker and cover. Cook on low for 8-12 hours or until lentils are tender. Stir in vinegar and mustard just before serving. Make sandwiches using toasted buns.

Southern Chickpeas and Grits

Ingredients:
1 green bell pepper, chopped
4 cloves garlic, minced
3 cups cooked chickpeas
1 cup water
3 cups diced tomatoes
1 tsp chipotle powder
3-4 dashes of liquid smoke
3-4 dashes of hot sauce
Salt and pepper to taste

Directions:
Combine all ingredients in the slow cooker and cook on low for 6-8 hours. Serve over a warm bowl of grits.

Lemon Pepper Tofu

Ingredients:
2 containers firm or extra firm tofu, pressed
3 TBSP brown sugar

2 TBSP soy sauce
1 TBSP apple cider vinegar
1 TBSP red pepper flakes
1/2 tsp garlic powder
1 ½ tsp lemon pepper
Juice from 1 lemon
Salt and pepper to taste

Directions:

Combine all ingredients in a slow cooker. Cover and cook on low for 5-6 hours.

No Beans Refried Beans

Ingredients:
2 medium butternut squash, peeled, seeded, and diced
1 cup sun dried tomatoes
1 TBSP tomato paste
1 cup water
2 tsp cumin
1 tsp cayenne
1 tsp chili powder
1 tsp garlic
Salt and pepper to taste

Directions:
Soak the tomatoes in water for half an hour. Place the tomatoes in the slow cooker and add in squash, tomato paste, sun dried tomatoes, and water. Sprinkle spices

on top and stir. Cook on low for 3 hours. Use a potato masher to create the consistency of refried beans.

Carrot Pudding

Ingredients:
4 large carrots, grated
1 small onion, grated
1/2 tsp Salt
1/4 tsp nutmeg
1 TBSP raw honey
1 cup almond milk
1 ½ bananas, pureed

Directions:
Mix together the carrots, onion, Salt, nutmeg, sugar, milk, and bananas. Pour into greased slow cooker; cover and cook on high for 3-4 hours.

Orange Pecan Carrots

Ingredients:
3 cups sliced carrots
3 TBSP coconut oil
2 cups water
3 TBSP organic orange jam
¼ tsp Salt
1/8 cup chopped pecans

Directions:
Combine all ingredients in the slow cooker and cover. Cook on low for 4-6 hours or until tender.

German Cole Slaw

Ingredients:
1 head cabbage, shredded
1 large onion, chopped
2 green peppers, chopped
1 tsp celery seed
1 ½ cups white vinegar
1 ½ tsp mustard seed
1 tsp turmeric
1 tsp Salt

Directions:
Combine all ingredients in the slow cooker and stir to make sure everything is thoroughly mixed. Cover and cook on low for 4-5 hours. Pour into a bowl and chill in refrigerator for at least 1 hour before serving.

Cauliflower Mash

Ingredients:
1 head of cauliflower, chopped
1 cup vegetable broth

2 TBSP coconut oil
Salt and pepper to taste

Directions:
Add cauliflower, vegetable broth, and coconut oil to slow cooker. Cook on low for 4 hours or until cauliflower is soft. Use a potato masher to mash cauliflower well and add Salt and pepper to taste.

Brocolli with Toasted Hazelnuts

Ingredients:
2 lbs. broccoli florets
1 cup of hazelnuts
1 TBSP olive oil
Juice from 2 lemons
½ tsp salt
½ tsp pepper

Directions:
Combine all ingredients in the slow cooker and toss to combine. Cover and cook on low for 4-5 hours or until broccoli reaches desired consistency.

Teriyaki Broccoli and Mushrooms

Ingredients:
2 cups broccoli florets
2 cups mushrooms, sliced

½ cup teriyaki sauce
½ cup pineapple juice
1 TBSP olive oil
½ tsp salt
½ tsp pepper

Directions:
Combine all ingredients in the slow cooker and toss to combine. Cover and cook on low for 4-5 hours or until broccoli reaches desired consistency.

Honey Dijon Brussels Sprouts

Ingredients:
1 pound Brussels sprouts
3 TBSP olive oil
1 TBSP Dijon mustard
¼ tsp salt
¼ tsp pepper
¼ cup water

Directions:
Combine all ingredients in the slow cooker and toss to combine. Cover and cook on low for 4-5 hours or until brussels sprouts reach desired consistency.

Lemon Pepper Brussels Sprouts

Ingredients:

1 pound Brussels sprouts
3 TBSP olive oil
Juice from 2 lemons
¼ tsp Salt
1 tsp lemon pepper
¼ cup water

Directions:
Combine all ingredients in the slow cooker and toss to combine. Cover and cook on low for 4-5 hours or until brussels sprouts reach desired consistency.

Garlic Lemon Asparagus

Ingredients:
1 pound asparagus spears, ends trimmed off
2 cloves garlic, minced
Juice from 1 lemon
1 TBSP olive oil
Salt and pepper to taste

Directions:
Combine all ingredients in the slow cooker and toss to combine. Cover and cook on low for around 2 hours or until tender crisp.

Winter Root Vegetable Medley

Ingredients:

2 pounds carrots
2 pounds rutabagas
2 pounds parsnips
½ cup chopped parsley
3 TBSP olive oil
1 tsp salt
1 tsp pepper
1 tsp basil

Directions:
Peel all the vegetables and cut into bite size chunks. Then toss into the slow cooker and combine with remaining ingredients. Cover and cook on low for 8-9 hours.

Smashed Turnips

Ingredients:
4 turnips, peeled and quartered
4 potatoes, peeled and quartered
2 TBSP minced onion
1 ½ tsp Salt, divided
Water
¼ cup cashew cream
2 TBSP olive oil
1/8 tsp pepper

Directions:
Combine turnips, potatoes, onions and 1 tsp of the Salt in the bottom of a slow cooker. Add water to cover.

Cover slow cooker and cook on low for 6-8 hours. Drain. Mash the mixture with a potato masher. Stir in remaining ingredients and continuing mashing until smooth.

Baked Sweet Potatoes

Ingredients:
5-6 Medium Sweet Potatoes
Salt and pepper to taste

Directions:
Wash sweet potatoes well but don't dry. Put on the bottom of the crock pot, put lid on, and turn on low. Cook for 6-8 hours or until tender. Serve with salt and pepper to taste.

Caramel Glazed Sweet Potatoes

Ingredients:
4 to 6 medium sweet potatoes, peeled and sliced
1 cup brown sugar
3 TBSP cornstarch
1 tsp cinnamon
½ tsp Salt
2 TBSP vegan butter spread

Directions:
Grease the slow cooker and add sliced sweet potatoes and sprinkle with Salt. Combine sugar, cornstarch and cinnamon; sprinkle over the sweet potatoes. Dot with Vegan butter spread; cover and cook on low for 7 to 9 hours.

Slow Cooker Corn on the Cob

Ingredients:
8 ears of corn
Olive Oil
Salt and pepper to taste

Directions:
Drizzle each ear of corn with olive oil and sprinkle on salt and pepper. Wrap in aluminum foil and place in the slow cooker. Once all ears are in the slow cooker, cover and cook on low for 4-5 hours or until corn is tender crisp.

Summer Garlic Green Beans

Ingredients:
1 pound green beans, washed and trimmed
2 TBSP olive oil
1 tsp Salt
¼ tsp pepper

3 cloves garlic, minced
1 cup vegetable broth

Directions:
Combine all ingredients in the slow cooker and toss to combine. Cover and cook on low for around 2 hours or until tender crisp.

Fast and Easy Slow Cooker Rice

Ingredients:
1 cup rice
2 cups water
Salt to taste
2 tsp olive oil

Directions:
Grease the slow cooker and pour in rice and water. Cover and cook on high for 1 ½ to 2 ½ hours, stirring occasionally.

Cajun Beans and Rice

Ingredients:
3 cups cooked beans
1 cup brown rice
1 cup vegetable broth
1 can of diced tomatoes
1 TBSP coconut oil, melted

1 tsp cumin
½ tsp garlic powder
2 cups water
½ cup Diced green chilies
Hot sauce or cayenne pepper to taste
Salt and pepper to taste

Directions:
Grease the slow cooker and pour in all ingredients. Cover and cook on high for 1 ½ to 2 ½ hours, stirring occasionally.

Sweet Pineapple Baked Beans

Ingredients:
2 cans pinto beans
1 8 ounce can pineapple chunks, drained
1 onion, diced
2 cloves garlic, minced
1/2 cup barbecue sauce
2 TBSP maple syrup
1 TBSP soy sauce
Salt and pepper to taste

Directions:
Combine all ingredients in the slow cooker and toss to combine. Cover and cook on low for around 6-8 hours.

Scalloped Potatoes

Ingredients:
1/2 onion, diced
2 cloves garlic, minced
1 TBSP parsley
1 tsp Salt
Pepper to taste
7-8 potatoes, sliced thin
8 oz Tofutti cream cheese substitute

Directions:
Lightly grease a slow cooker. In a small bowl, combine the onion, garlic, parsley, Salt, and pepper. Place a layer of the sliced potatoes on the bottom of the slow cooker. Sprinkle with some of the onion and garlic mix. Top with 1/3 of the Tofutti. Continue layering potatoes, spices and cream cheese. Sprinkle the top with additional Salt and pepper. Cover and cook on high for 3-4 hours, or until potatoes are done cooking.

Vegan Slow Cooker Fudge

Ingredients:
2 ½ cups Vegan chocolate chips
½ cup canned coconut milk
¼ cup honey
1/8 tsp Salt
1 tsp pure vanilla extract
Coconut oil

Directions:
Grease the slow cooker with coconut oil. In a bowl, stir together all ingredients except vanilla and then pour into the slow cooker. Cook on high for 2 hours. Uncover and turn off heat; stir in vanilla extract. Then leave the mixture uncovered in the slow cooker (turned off) for 3-4 hours until it's room temperature. When it reaches room temperature, stir for 10 minutes and then pour into a well-greased container and cool in the fridge overnight.

Bananas Foster

Ingredients:
4 bananas, medium firmness
1 TBSP coconut oil
1 TBSP lemon juice
3 TBSP raw honey
1 tsp cinnamon
½ tsp nutmeg
½ tsp cloves

Directions:

Combine all ingredients except bananas into slow cooker and turn on high for 5-10 minutes or until melted. Stir together and then reduce slow cooker heat to low. Slice bananas to ¼ inch thick and add them in the slow cooker. Toss to combine with honey mixture. Cook on low for 2 hours.

Honey Glazed Pears

Ingredients:
4 pears, halved and cored
1 TBSP lemon juice
1 cup raw honey
2 TBSp coconut oil, melted
¼ cup water
½ tsp pure vanilla extra
1 tsp cinnamon

Directions:
Place pears in your slow cooker and top with remaining ingredients. Stir together gently to combine. Cover and cook on low for 4-6 hours or until pears are fork tender.

Southern Cherry Jubilee

Ingredients:
2 TBSP melted coconut oil
4 cups black cherries, pitted
1 cup raw honey
Zest from ½ lemon
1 cup water
½ tsp cinnamon

Directions:

Combine all ingredients in a slow cooker and cover. Cook on low for 3-4 hours. Serve with whipped coconut cream if desired.

Walnut Strawberry Surprise

Ingredients:
3 cups fresh strawberries, capped and quartered
½ cup honey
1 tsp cinnamon
1 tsp pure maple syrup
½ cup walnuts, chopped
1 cup water
Zest from ½ lemon

Directions:
Combine all ingredients in your slow cooker and toss to mix. Cover and cook on low for 3-4 hours.

Hawaiian Tapioca Pudding

Ingredients:
¾ cup raw honey
1 cup small pearl tapioca
3 cups coconut milk
1 egg

½ cup coconut
½ cup chopped pineapple

Directions:
Combine all ingredients and pour into a well greased slow cooker. Cover and cook on low for 4 hours.

Berry Mint Medley

Ingredients:
1 cup blackberries
1 cup blueberries
1 cup raspberries
½ cup raw honey
½ cup coconut milk
1 tsp allspice
Small handful fresh mint, chopped

Directions:

Combine all ingredients except for mint in the slow cooker. Stir and cover. Cook on low for 2 hours. Add in mint leaves and cook for another 30 minutes.

Chocolate Peanut Butter Cake

Ingredients:
Cake:

1 cup flour
½ cup sugar
2 TBSP cocoa powder
1 ½ tsp baking powder
½ cup soy milk
2 TBSP coconut oil, melted
1 tsp vanilla
¾ cup vegan chocolate chips

Peanut Butter Layer:
¾ cup sugar
¼ cup cocoa powder
1 cup boiling water
½ cup peanut butter

Directions:
Grease the slow cooker. In a mixing bowl, combine the cake ingredients and mix until smooth. Pour into the prepared slow cooker. In a mixing bowl, combine the sugar and cocoa powder. In a separate bowl, combine the boiling water and the peanut butter. Mix into the cocoa mixture.

Carefully pour evenly over the cake batter. Cover and cook on high for 2 to 2 ½ hours, until a toothpick inserted into the center comes out clean.

Simple Rice Pudding

Ingredients:

4 cups vanilla soy milk
1 cup uncooked rice
1 cup sugar
3 TBSP Vegan margarine
Pinch of Salt
1 tsp vanilla
¼ cup dried cranberries
¼ cup raisins
½ tsp cinnamon

Directions:
Combine all the ingredients in a slow cooker. Cook on low for 2 to 4 hours, stirring every hour, until the desired consistency is reached.

Slow Cooker Apple Cobbler

Ingredients:
4 ½ cups granny smith apples, peeled, cored, and sliced
2 TBSP flour
1/3 cup white sugar
¾ cup brown sugar
1/3 cup dried cranberries
¼ tsp cinnamon
2/3 cup oats
1 cup water
3 TBSP melted Vegan margarine

Directions:
In a mixing bowl, toss the apples in the flour and white sugar to coat. Stir in the dried cranberries, cinnamon, and oats. Pour the water into a slow cooker and add the apple mixture. Pour the melted Vegan margarine over the apples and sprinkle with the brown sugar. Cover and cook on low for 4 to 6 hours, or until the apples are tender.

Georgia Peach Cobbler

Ingredients:
4 ½ cups sliced peaches
2 TBSP flour
1/3 cup white sugar
¾ cup brown sugar
½ tsp cinnamon
2/3 cup oats
1 cup water
3 TBSP melted Vegan margarine

Directions:
In a mixing bowl, toss the peaches in the flour and white sugar to coat. Stir in the cinnamon and oats. Pour the water into a slow cooker and add the peach mixture. Pour the melted Vegan margarine over the apples and sprinkle with the brown sugar. Cover and cook on low for 4 to 6 hours, or until the peaches are tender.

Crustless Pumpkin Pie

Ingredients:
15-oz. can pumpkin
1 1/3 cups nondairy creamer
½ cup sugar
¼ cup brown sugar
½ cup Bisquick
Egg replacer equivalent to 2 eggs
2 TBSP melted Vegan margarine
2 ½ tsp pumpkin pie spice
2 tsp vanilla

Directions:
Combine all ingredients in a bowl and pour into a greased slow cooker. Cook on low for 7-8 hours.

Apple Pudding Can Cake

Ingredients:
2 cups sugar
1 cup vegetable oil
Egg replacer equivalent to 2 eggs
2 tsp vanilla
2 cups flour
1 tsp baking soda
1 tsp nutmeg
2 cups unpeeled apple, finely chopped
1 cup chopped nuts (walnuts or pecans)

Directions:
Beat together sugar, oil, egg substitute, and vanilla. Add apple with dry ingredients and mix well. Take a 2-pound tin can and grease well. Pour the cake batter into can, filling no more than 2/3 full. Place the can in your slow cooker and cover, but leave a gap for steam to escape. Cook on high for 3 ½ to 4 hours. Cake is done when the top is set.

Cherry Cobbler

Ingredients:
1 can cherry pie filling
2/3 cup brown sugar
½ cup quick-cooking oats
½ cup flour
1 tsp brown sugar
1/3 Vegan margarine butter, softened

Directions:
Grease the slow cooker and place cherry pie filling in the bottom. Combine dry ingredients in a mixing bowl and cut in margarine with a pastry cutter. Sprinkle crumbs over cherry filling. Cover and cook on low for 5 hours.

Simple Marinara Sauce

Ingredients:
- 2 (28 oz.) cans crushed tomatoes
- 1 (6 oz.) can tomato paste
- 1 medium yellow onion, chopped
- ½ TBSP minced garlic
- 2 whole bay leaves
- 1 TBSP Italian seasoning
- 1 TBSP brown sugar
- 1 TBSP balsamic vinegar

Salt and pepper to taste

Directions:
Combine all ingredients in the slow cooker and cover. Cook on low for 8-10 hours.

www.ingramcontent.com/pod-product-compliance
Lightning Source LLC
Chambersburg PA
CBHW071441070526
44578CB00001B/182